Clinical Diagnostic Tests

Clinical Diagnostic Tests

How to Avoid Errors in Ordering Tests and Interpreting Results

Edited by

Michael Laposata, MD, PhD
Professor and Chair
Department of Pathology
University of Texas Medical Branch–Galveston
Galveston, Texas

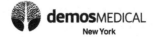

demosMEDICAL
New York

Visit our website at www.demosmedical.com

ISBN: 9781620700839
e-book ISBN: 9781617052620

Acquisitions Editor: Rich Winters
Compositor: diacriTech

Medicine is an ever-changing science. Research and clinical experience are continually expanding our knowledge, in particular our understanding of proper treatment and drug therapy. The authors, editors, and publisher have made every effort to ensure that all information in this book is in accordance with the state of knowledge at the time of production of the book. Nevertheless, the authors, editors, and publisher are not responsible for errors or omissions or for any consequences from application of the information in this book and make no warranty, expressed or implied, with respect to the contents of the publication. Every reader should examine carefully the package inserts accompanying each drug and should carefully check whether the dosage schedules mentioned therein or the contraindications stated by the manufacturer differ from the statements made in this book. Such examination is particularly important with drugs that are either rarely used or have been newly released on the market.

Library of Congress Cataloging-in-Publication Data
Clinical diagnostic tests : how to avoid errors in ordering tests and interpreting results / editor, Michael Laposata.
  p. ; cm.
  Includes bibliographical references and index.
  ISBN 978-1-62070-083-9—ISBN 978-1-61705-262-0 (ebook)
  I. Laposata, Michael, editor.
  [DNLM: 1. Clinical Laboratory Techniques—methods. 2. Diagnostic Tests, Routine—methods. 3. Diagnostic Errors—prevention & control. WB 200]
  RC71.2
  616.07'5—dc23

                              2015016835

Special discounts on bulk quantities of Demos Medical Publishing books are available to corporations, professional associations, pharmaceutical companies, health care organizations, and other qualifying groups. For details, please contact:

Special Sales Department
Demos Medical Publishing, LLC
11 West 42nd Street, 15th Floor
New York, NY 10036
Phone: 800-532-8663 or 212-683-0072
Fax: 212-941-7842
E-mail: specialsales@demosmedical.com

Printed in the United States of America by Gasch.
14 15 16 17 / 5 4 3 2 1

Contents

Contributors   *vii*
Preface   *ix*

1. Transfusion Medicine   *1*
Quentin G. Eichbaum, Garrett S. Booth, and
Pampee P. Young

2. Coagulation Disorders   *59*
Michael Laposata

3. Hematology and Immunology   *121*
Adam C. Seegmiller and
Mary Ann Thompson Arildsen

4. Clinical Chemistry   *143*
James H. Nichols and Carol A. Rauch

5. Clinical Microbiology   *191*
Charles W. Stratton

6. Laboratory Management   *259*
Candis A. Kinkus

Index   *287*

Contributors

Mary Ann Thompson Arildsen, MD, PhD
Department of Pathology, Microbiology and
  Immunology
Vanderbilt University School of Medicine
Nashville, Tennessee

Garrett S. Booth, MD, MS
Department of Pathology, Microbiology and
  Immunology
Vanderbilt University School of Medicine
Nashville, Tennessee

**Quentin G. Eichbaum, MD, PhD, MPH, MFA,
  MMHC, FCAP**
Department of Pathology, Microbiology and
  Immunology
Vanderbilt University School of Medicine
Nashville, Tennessee

Candis A. Kinkus, MBA
Diagnostic Laboratories
Vanderbilt University Medical Center
Nashville, Tennessee

Michael Laposata, MD, PhD
Department of Pathology
University of Texas Medical Branch–Galveston
Galveston, Texas

James H. Nichols, PhD, DABCC, FACB
Department of Pathology, Microbiology and
    Immunology
Vanderbilt University School of Medicine
Nashville, Tennessee

Carol A. Rauch, MD, PhD, FCAP
Department of Pathology, Microbiology and
    Immunology
Vanderbilt University School of Medicine
Nashville, Tennessee

Adam C. Seegmiller, MD, PhD
Department of Pathology, Microbiology and
    Immunology
Vanderbilt University School of Medicine
Nashville, Tennessee

Charles W. Stratton, MD
Department of Pathology, Microbiology and
    Immunology
Vanderbilt University School of Medicine
Nashville, Tennessee

Pampee P. Young, MD, PhD
Department of Pathology, Microbiology and
    Immunology; and
Department of Medicine
Vanderbilt University School of Medicine
Nashville, Tennessee

Preface

The Institute of Medicine in the United States has recently organized a committee, of which I am a member, on diagnostic error in health care. It has become clear that major contributors to diagnostic mistakes include the incorrect selection of laboratory tests and the misinterpretation of laboratory test results. As the clinical laboratory test menu has greatly expanded in the past decade in size, complexity, and cost, the challenge of ordering the right tests, and only the right tests, and correctly interpreting complex test results, has become a significant challenge for most health care providers for a larger and larger percentage of their patients.

The idea to produce books describing medical errors related to inappropriate selection of laboratory tests and misinterpretation of laboratory test results first emerged in a discussion in a restaurant in Chicago. The first challenge was to determine whose medical errors would be reported. Would this be a compilation of medical errors reported in the literature, personally observed medical errors in the experience of an author, or admissions of unpublished mistakes by medical colleagues? Ultimately, it was decided to invite established experts in the different areas of laboratory medicine to become authors who could bring forward errors that they had read about, personally encountered, or learned from discussions with clinical and laboratory colleagues. The goal for each author was to identify and describe the most common mistakes in his or her specialty area of laboratory medicine, and then use those mistakes to create a set of "standards of care" that would lead to a reduction in the frequency of those errors. Six separate books were produced in the series, and they describe errors in laboratory testing for coagulation, transfusion medicine, clinical chemistry, clinical microbiology, hematology and immunology, and the often overlooked area of laboratory management. The organization of each book is similar. A major group of diagnostic errors associated with the clinical laboratory (such as those in which an abscess is mistakenly concluded to be a malignancy because of findings in the microbiology laboratory) is introduced with a brief background on that group of medical errors, followed by an actual case to illustrate this error, then a short statement that describes the clinical pitfall, and finally a list of standards of care related to, in this example, appropriate testing to minimize the number of cases mistakenly identified as abscesses that are, in fact, malignancies. After production of the last of the six books, it was recognized that removal of the case examples would allow all six books to be combined into the one clinically valuable book which follows this preface.

It is with great hope that this book, which identifies medical errors associated with laboratory testing, will be useful in the education of medical students, interns and residents in all medical fields, clinical laboratory technologists, and practicing physicians—so that they may learn from the mistakes of others and not make new mistakes of their own. If the specific errors described in this book were all reduced in frequency by more than 90%, there would be a tremendous improvement in patient outcome and a substantial reduction in the cost of health care.

Michael Laposata, MD, PhD

CHAPTER 1
Transfusion Medicine

QUENTIN G. EICHBAUM
GARRETT S. BOOTH
PAMPEE P. YOUNG

PRODUCT-RELATED ERRORS

INAPPROPRIATE USE OF FRESH FROZEN PLASMA TO CORRECT MILDLY ELEVATED PROTHROMBIN TIME

In patients scheduled for minimally invasive surgical procedures, whose prothrombin time (PT) or international normalized ratio (INR) is only slightly elevated, the concern for significant bleeding may be unwarranted, and there is generally no need to transfuse fresh frozen plasma (FFP) to replenish coagulation factors. When the PT/INR is only mildly elevated, infusion of FFP to replenish coagulation factors will have little impact on further lowering the PT/INR, due to the physiologic reserve of these coagulation factors.

Patients may be unnecessarily transfused with FFP in an attempt to decrease a slightly elevated PT/INR back into the normal range. Such transfusion of FFP may, moreover, have the unwanted consequence of precipitating an adverse event in the form of a transfusion reaction. Potential adverse events to transfusion of FFP include volume overload, allergic reactions, transfusion-related lung injury, and transmission of infectious agents.

Clinical Pitfall

Failure to recognize that coagulation screening tests can be poor predictors of bleeding and that use of FFP to lower a minimally elevated PT into the normal range may be counterproductive.

STANDARDS OF CARE

- Coagulation screening test results should not be too conservatively interpreted, but should be assessed in the setting of the hemostatic defect, the patient's underlying condition, the procedure to be performed, and the likelihood of bleeding.
- A slightly elevated PT/INR (12–17 seconds; INR 1.0–1.7) is usually not a cause for concern in a patient undergoing a minimally invasive or bedside procedure, who is not bleeding, and who has no history of excess bleeding or bruising.

INAPPROPRIATE USE OF FFP FOR VOLUME EXPANSION

Plasma is used primarily for the purpose of preventing bleeding and to treat hemorrhage in patients with acquired or congenital coagulation defects. Besides FFP, other plasma products are also available, including plasma frozen within 24 hours of phlebotomy (FP24), which is often used interchangeably with FFP; thawed plasma (derived from FFP or FP24 that has been thawed and kept at 1°C–6°C and can be stored for up to five days); and cryoprecipitate-reduced plasma that consists of the supernatant that is removed when cryoprecipitate is made from FFP.

Appropriate indications for the use of plasma products include coagulation factor replacement in congenital factor defects where factor concentrates are unavailable, massive transfusion, plasma exchange transfusions, reversal of warfarin anticoagulation in the setting of severe bleeding, and treatment of disseminated intravascular coagulation. Plasma products should not be used for volume expansion, as a source of nutrients, to treat immunodeficiency, or to promote wound healing. As with other blood products, administration of plasma products may be associated with adverse reactions, so nonmedically indicated usage should be carefully avoided.

Clinical Pitfall

Failure to understand the appropriate clinical usage of plasma products.

STANDARDS OF CARE

- Volume depletion should generally be treated with normal saline or crystalloid, and not with plasma or other blood products.
- Plasma products should be used to prevent bleeding or to treat acquired and congenital coagulation defects.

INAPPROPRIATE USE OF Rh IMMUNE GLOBULIN IN PREGNANCY

The use of pooled, human-derived immunoglobulins directed against the RhD antigen (Rh immune globulin [RhIG]) is a success story of modern immunohematology and obstetrics. Prior to the 1970s, hemolytic disease of the fetus and newborn (HDFN) was a common clinical problem, with considerable neonatal morbidity and mortality. Previous treatments, including exchange transfusions and phototherapy, were both risky and financially cumbersome. With the advent of routine prophylactic administration of RhIG at 28 to 30 weeks gestation, and again at the conclusion of pregnancy, alloimmunization to RhD decreased by 90%, as did the incidence of HDFN.

Clinical Pitfall

Failure to recognize the appropriate use of RhIG.

STANDARDS OF CARE

■ Both American Association of Blood Banks (AABB) and American Congress of Obstetricians and Gynecologists (ACOG) recommend routine ABO/Rh typing of pregnant females, with additional intervention at 28 to 30 weeks for those patients who type as Rh-negative and with a negative antibody screen.

■ Additional RhIG should be administered at the time of delivery, or in cases where the fetal–maternal blood barrier has been disrupted (ie, amniocentesis).

RhIG—INADEQUATE DOSING

Pregnant Rh-negative females, carrying an Rh-positive baby, who experience a fetomaternal hemorrhage (FMH) of even just a few milliliters of blood, are at increased risk for alloimmunization to the RhD antigen unless they receive an adequate dose of RhIG. The volume of blood causing anti-D alloimmunization varies among patients and appears to be related to factors such as the immunologic responsiveness of the mother and the immunogenicity of the Rh-positive red blood cells (RBCs). The rosette test serves as the initial screen for the presence of FMH. The volume of FMH (percentage of fetal red cells in the maternal circulation) is then determined by the Kleihauer–Betke test (an acid elution test) or, more precisely and reliably, by flow cytometry. Combinations of these tests can also be used to identify and quantify such hemorrhage.

RhIG provides prophylaxis to prevent alloimmunization to the RhD blood group antigen in Rh-negative patients exposed to Rh-positive RBCs during transfusion, placental bleeding, or pregnancy. The mechanism of action of RhIG remains unclear, but the correct level of dosing has been empirically determined and is important to prevent alloimmunization.

The appropriate dose of RhIG is determined by a calculation that takes into account the percentage of fetal RBCs in the maternal circulation and the mother's blood volume. Inadequate dosing of RhIG may fail to protect the mother from anti-D alloimmunization, which may result in hemolytic disease of the newborn in subsequent pregnancies.

Clinical Pitfall

Failure to correctly assess the amount of FMH and to administer the appropriate dose of RhIG prophylaxis to avert anti-D alloimmunization in an Rh-negative mother carrying an Rh-positive fetus.

STANDARDS OF CARE

- When FMH occurs during routine delivery, or is suspected as a consequence of placental bleeding, a sample of maternal blood should be collected for FMH testing within an hour of the event.
- The rosette test is performed to screen for FMH and, if positive, is succeeded by either the Kleihauer–Betke test or, preferably, by the more sensitive flow cytometric testing, to quantify the volume of FMH.
- The dose of RhIG administered to the mother is calculated by giving 300 mcg vial doses of RhIG per 30 mL of fetal whole blood, or per 15 mL of fetal RBCs, in the maternal circulation. (Note: other dose sizes of RhIG are also available.)

Calculation for RhIG dosing:

- ✓ Maternal blood volume (mL) = 70 mL/kg × maternal weight (kg) [*use 5,000 mL if maternal weight is not known*]
- ✓ Volume of fetal bleed (mL) = Percentage of fetal RBCs × maternal blood volume

✓ Dose of RhIG (300 mcg vials) to administer = fetal bleed (mL)/30 mL of whole blood (*or 15 mL of RBCs*)

✓ If the number to the right of the decimal point is less than 5, round the number down and add one additional dose of RhIG (eg, 3.4 → 3 + 1 = 4); if the number to the right of the decimal greater than 5, round up and add an additional dose of RhIG (eg, 2.8 → 3 + 1 = 4).

INAPPROPRIATE USE OF CRYOPRECIPITATE

The appropriate use of cryoprecipitate is highly variable. In part, this is due to a misunderstanding of what this blood product contains. However, there is also a dearth of evidence from randomized controlled trials about appropriate usage. Its indiscriminate usage, as evident from numerous blood bank audits, appears to be driven by the misguided belief that it represents a "super concentrated" form of FFP. This is not true, as cryoprecipitate has a different composition than FFP.

Clinical Pitfall

Failure to recognize the appropriate usage of cryoprecipitate and to calculate the correct dose.

STANDARDS OF CARE

■ As per American Association of Blood Banks (AABB) *Standards*, cryoprecipitate contains specified amounts per unit of fibrinogen (minimum of 150 mg) and factor VIII (minimum 80 IU). It also contains factor XIII (40–60 IU), von Willebrand Factor (~80 IU), and fibronectin (40–60 IU). It is used primarily in the control of bleeding associated with fibrinogen deficiency and in the treatment of factor XIII deficiency, but can also be used as a second-line therapy for von Willebrand disease and hemophilia A.

The number of unit bags of fibrinogen to administer, based on level of fibrinogen desired, is calculated as follows:

1. Calculate the total blood volume:
   - Body weight (kg) × 70 mL/kg
2. Calculate the total plasma volume:
   - Total blood volume × (1 – hematocrit)
3. Calculate the milligrams of fibrinogen needed:
   - (Total plasma volume) × (concentration change in fibrinogen desired):
     - The change in fibrinogen level desired is determined by subtracting the current level from the desired level of fibrinogen; for example, if the desired level is 175 mg/dL and the current fibrinogen level is 50 mg/dL: 175 – 50 mg/dL = 125 mg/dL
   - Multiply the change in concentration times the total plasma volume, but divide the answer by 100 to correct the units (dL to mL)
4. Calculate the number of bags needed to reach the desired fibrinogen level:
   - Number of bags needed/150 mg per bag

PLATELET INACTIVATION AS A RESULT OF COLD EXPOSURE

Whole blood and blood components must be stored and handled in accordance with regulatory standards to maintain therapeutic potency and ensure the safety of patients. Whereas packed red cells and plasma are stored and transported at cold temperatures (ranging from 1°C to 6°C), platelets are required to be maintained at room temperature, between 20°C and 24°C. Exposure of platelets, even briefly, to temperatures under 15°C renders them inactive and unsuitable for clinical use.

Clinical Pitfall

Failure to keep platelet products at appropriate temperature.

STANDARDS OF CARE

- Platelets should be issued in a specialized bag with a label warning not to expose them to cold temperatures or ice.
- The transfusion service should educate hospital providers about appropriate temperatures for keeping platelets.
- Platelets that are exposed to cold must be discarded because such exposure targets them in vivo for destruction by liver and spleen macrophages following transfusion.

ERRORS IN PROCEDURES

A POSITIVE TYPE AND SCREEN WILL RESULT IN RELATIVE DELAY IN THE ISSUE OF BLOOD

Timely issue and delivery of RBCs are critical to optimal patient care. Experienced surgeons often have some estimates of expected blood loss for a given procedure. In many institutions, surgeons request RBCs to be packed in a validated "cooler" prior to the start of surgery based on these estimated blood losses. However, surgical outcome can be quite variable, and bleeding is often unanticipated. This inherent uncertainty and complexity in surgical practice underscores the importance of the reliable and timely release of blood products from the blood bank.

In order to issue crossmatched RBC products, the blood bank must have verified the patient's blood type and must have tested the patient's plasma to determine whether any non-ABO RBC antibodies are present (eg, D, Kell, and Jka). If the screen is negative, RBCs can be issued with an immediate spin crossmatch (which takes a few minutes to perform manually) or an electronic crossmatch (performed in less time by computer verification of the patient's blood type and the absence of any antibodies in plasma). Most clinicians, including surgeons, assume that RBCs can be obtained immediately when the screen is negative. When the screen is positive, the crossmatch process is more involved and requires at least an hour to complete.

Clinical Pitfall

Failure to anticipate a potential delay in the issue of blood based on the patient's blood type and screen result.

STANDARDS OF CARE

- Two units of crossmatched RBCs should be on reserve for each patient scheduled for surgery who has a positive antibody screen.
- The clinical team should be notified by the blood bank whenever there is an anticipated delay in providing crossmatch-compatible units.

ERROR IN BLOOD SAMPLE COLLECTION RESULTING IN INACCURATE TYPE AND SCREEN

The location and manner in which a blood sample is collected for laboratory testing may be a source of significant medical error. For instance, a blood sample collected from a heparin-flushed line may show an elevated partial thromboplastin time (PTT). A blood sample collected from a vein in the same extremity and "upstream" from a vein into which blood is being transfused will likely yield inaccurate laboratory results as it will be mixed with transfused blood.

Clinical Pitfall

Failure to recognize the importance of correct blood sampling technique for blood typing.

STANDARDS OF CARE

■ Samples for a type and screen assay should not be collected from a vein proximal to the site where donor blood is simultaneously being transfused in a patient.

■ Specimens received by blood bank laboratories must at a minimum have the correct patient information on the label, including, but not limited to, patient last name, patient first name, date, time, and phlebotomist identification.

MISINTERPRETATION OF LABORATORY TESTS FOR HEMOLYSIS

In emergency transfusions, there is typically no time to perform a patient's blood type and screen, and therefore universal donor group O Rh-negative RBCs are transfused. The major concern is to maintain the patient's blood oxygen carrying capacity by monitoring the hemoglobin (Hgb)/hematocrit levels, and to prevent symptomatic anemia.

Without an antibody screen, the potential risk exists for a delayed hemolytic transfusion reaction in patients who have been alloimmunized to minor RBC antigens. Such hemolysis could lead to a worsening anemia. Usually, but not always, out-of-group transfusions have clinical consequences. However, in massive transfusions, when the equivalent of more than a total adult blood volume of blood is not screened for reactivity against clinically significant antigens, the risk of delayed hemolytic reactions (DHTRs) increases due to the exposure to large amounts of donor blood.

Hemolytic reactions may be identified by a panel of laboratory tests that can include a lactate dehydrogenase (LDH) level, bilirubin (total, direct, indirect), liver enzymes (aspartate aminotransferase, AST; alanine aminotransferase, ALT), the reticulocyte count, a haptoglobin level, and a peripheral blood smear.

Numerous medical conditions other than hemolysis, especially hepatorenal and cardiac conditions, are associated with abnormalities in these test values. In the setting of transfusion, failure to take into account other underlying comorbidities affecting these test values can lead to the erroneous conclusion that RBC hemolysis has occurred.

Clinical Pitfall

Failure to recognize that elevated LDH, bilirubin, and haptoglobin values do not always indicate RBC hemolysis but may be associated with other underlying comorbidities.

STANDARDS OF CARE

- A negative antibody screen and direct antiglobulin test (DAT) in a patient with a history of alloimmunization reduces the likelihood of a DHTR.
- Alternate comorbidities should be considered in interpreting laboratory test values typically used in the evaluation for RBC lysis (eg, LDH, bilirubin, and haptoglobin).
- A peripheral blood smear should be examined to check for immune hemolysis.

ABO TYPING DISCREPANCY DUE TO LESS COMMON ABO SUBGROUPS

A blood type is based on the presence or absence of inherited antigenic structures on the surface of RBCs. The ABO system is the most important blood group system in human blood transfusion. The associated anti-A and anti-B antibodies are both class IgM and IgG immunoglobulins. ABO IgM and IgG antibodies are produced in the first years of life, probably as a result of sensitization to environmental substances, such as food, bacteria, and viruses. ABO typing involves both antigen typing and antibody detection.

The antigen typing is referred to as the forward typing, and the antibody detection is the reverse typing.

Clinical Pitfall

Failure to recognize minor ABO subgroups and their clinical significance.

STANDARDS OF CARE

■ Failure to properly type both the donor and recipient can result in life-threatening harm to the recipient. It also represents poor management of heart organs suitable for transplantation, a rare and valuable resource.

INAPPROPRIATE USE OF AUTOLOGOUS BLOOD

It is estimated that almost half of all blood transfusions performed in the United States occur perioperatively. What is often not realized is that there are several alternatives to the transfusion of allogeneic blood. The most common alternatives include intraoperative blood salvage, acute normovolemic hemodilution, and transfusion with banked autologous blood. Each of these alternatives, however, carries advantages and disadvantages. Transfusion of autologous blood is no exception.

Clinical Pitfall

Failure to understand the appropriate use of autologous RBC transfusions.

STANDARDS OF CARE

■ Autologous blood donation should be performed prior to surgery to avoid unnecessary iatrogenic blood loss (minimum time >72 hours; optimal time frame is approximately one week prior to procedure).

AABB and FDA standards indicate that autologous donors should have an Hgb count of at least 11 g/dL (hematocrit 33%) and should be relatively healthy.

RAPID TRANSFUSION IN CHRONIC ANEMIA MAY RESULT IN VOLUME OVERLOAD

Children and adults with severe chronic anemia (Hgb <5.0 g/dL) are usually transfused slowly in order to reduce the risk of transfusion-associated circulatory overload (TACO). Patients with severe chronic anemia have a relatively normal circulating blood volume (70–80 mL/kg), but with a compensatory increase in their plasma volume that increases their risk for TACO.

Clinical Pitfall

Failure to recognize the increased risk of TACO in patients with chronic anemia.

STANDARDS OF CARE

- A single unit of transfused blood product can be sufficient to cause TACO; vigilance for volume overload is required even with small volumes of transfused products.
- In pediatrics, if the Hgb is less than 5 g/dL, transfuse over a period of 4 hours the following calculated volume: *number of milliliters = Hgb × weight in kilograms.*

COLD AGGLUTININ DISEASE—INSIGNIFICANCE OF LOW ANTIBODY TITERS

Cold agglutinin disease (CAD) is caused by IgM autoantibodies that can agglutinate RBCs in vitro at cold temperatures (4°C–18°C). These autoantibodies can cause intravascular hemolysis in vivo, especially when present in high titers at warmer temperatures (30°C–37°C). The hemolysis is mediated by the classic complement pathway that lyses the RBC membrane, releasing Hgb and resulting in hemoglobinemia, hemoglobinuria, and low free haptoglobin.

When the antibody concentration is not sufficiently high to activate the full complement cascade, complement activation is taken only to the C3 stage, producing RBCs coated with C3b without hemolysis. The titer and temperature at which hemolysis occurs can vary, but titers lower than 1 to 32 only rarely cause clinically significant hemolysis. Evidence suggests that only titers of autoantibody greater to 1 to 1,000 are clinically significant. When the antibody is not reactive at 30°C or higher, hemolysis is unlikely when the titers are low.

Clinical Pitfall

Failure to recognize that low titers of cold agglutinins can be detected in normal individuals and are only rarely clinically significant.

STANDARDS OF CARE

- In CAD, at low IgM antibody titers, only supportive treatment such as avoidance of cold temperatures, is necessary.
- The need for transfusion should be assessed by the degree of the anemia.

HYPOCALCEMIC TOXICITY FROM THERAPEUTIC PLASMA EXCHANGE

Hypocalcemic toxicity is one of the most common adverse effects of therapeutic plasma exchange (TPE). The symptoms of this toxicity are associated with a decrease in plasma ionized calcium. The normal range for total calcium concentration in the plasma is 8.5 to

10.5 mg/dL. Approximately 50% of this concentration is ionized, 40% is bound to proteins (primarily albumin), and 10% circulates in a form bound to anions. Citrate-based anticoagulants, notably sodium citrate, are a major cause of hypocalcemic toxicity as the citrate binds to and thereby lowers the intravascular ionized calcium levels. In addition, replacement fluids such as human albumin and FFP may contribute to hypocalcemia. It is important to recognize the signs and symptoms of hypocalcemic toxicity because effective interventions are readily available.

Clinical Pitfall

Failure to monitor and treat hypocalcemia during a therapeutic apheresis procedure that leads to hypocalcemic toxicity.

STANDARDS OF CARE

- Treatments of hypocalcemic toxicity should be appropriately implemented; these include slowing the infusion rate, providing calcium replacements (intravenous or oral), and/or adding calcium directly to replacement fluids such as albumin.
- For patients experiencing hypocalcemia, careful monitoring is required for life-threatening complications, such as laryngospasm or cardiac arrhythmias.

HEMOLYSIS FOLLOWING PLATELET TRANSFUSION

When ABO group-specific platelet concentrates are not available, it is common practice to transfuse ABO out-of-group platelets. An adult dose of platelets contains approximately 250 mL of donor plasma. Infusion of this plasma can result in the passive transfer of anti-A and/or anti-B antibodies. Usually, this does not result in any serologically evident or clinically significant hemolysis. Rarely, however, transfusion of out-of-group platelets can lead to significant passive alloimmune hemolysis due to "passively" transferred antibodies in the residual plasma in the product. Deaths have occurred due to such hemolysis attributable to transfusion of out-of-group platelets.

Clinical Pitfall

Failure to diagnose a passively mediated hemolytic transfusion reaction due to a minor incompatibility between donor plasma and recipient red cells.

STANDARDS OF CARE

- The recommendations of the National Blood Service Transfusion Medicine Clinical Policies Group are (a) platelets from donors with identical ABO group are the component of choice, (b) administration of ABO incompatible platelets is acceptable when platelets are in short supply, and (c) group O platelets should not be given if known to be a high titer for anti-A or anti-B isohemagglutinins.

DEVELOPMENT OF COAGULOPATHY SECONDARY TO INTENSIVE TPE

Plasmapheresis, or TPE, is the process by which whole blood is withdrawn from an individual's circulation, one of its components, such as plasma, is separated out, and the remainder of the blood is returned together with a replacement fluid. In therapy for some diseases, such as thrombotic thrombocytopenic purpura (TTP), the replacement fluid is plasma from healthy donors. In other diseases, such as myasthenia gravis (MG), the replacement fluid can be albumin or a combination of albumin and normal saline. Such replacement fluids have the benefit of avoiding exposure to donor plasma that may induce infectious and immunologic complications.

Clinical Pitfall

Failure to compensate for dilution of coagulation factors from plasmapheresis.

STANDARDS OF CARE

- Dilution of coagulation factors in procedures involving the removal of plasma must be assessed by the measurement of PT and PTT values before and after the procedure.
- Plasma exchange can also cause a decrease in platelets. Platelet counts should therefore also be monitored.

HEPARIN-FLUSHED LINES—INADVERTENT EXPOSURE TO BLOOD CIRCULATION

In apheresis procedures, the blood of a patient or donor is circulated through an apparatus that separates out one particular constituent for collection or therapeutic intervention, and returns the remainder of the components to the circulation. Extracorporeal photopheresis (ECP) is an apheresis procedure (used for instance in the treatment of graft versus host disease [GVHD]) in which the patient's white blood cells and platelets are separated out for treatment with photoactivating drugs and then exposed to ultraviolet light before being returned to the patient's circulation where they exert a therapeutic effect. Photopheresis instruments may be flushed with heparin (or citrate-containing solutions) as anticoagulants. As some patients may not tolerate heparin, a careful clinical history should be taken prior to commencing procedures that include this anticoagulant.

While a patient with known heparin-induced thrombocytopenia would be unlikely to be scheduled for procedures that use heparin, patients with less obvious underlying conditions associated with a risk for bleeding (such as subarachnoid hemorrhage) may fail to be excluded. Such patients may inadvertently be exposed to heparin in different ways. There is a tendency to regard the flushing of instrument lines with heparin as standard practice and innocuous to patients. Yet serious complications, such as drug interactions, iatrogenic hemorrhage, and heparin-induced thrombocytopenia, have been reported in association with such heparin flushing.

If heparin is contraindicated for patients, citrate contained in solutions such as acid-citrate-dextrose formula A can be used as an anticoagulant.

Clinical Pitfall

Failure (averted) to recognize that apheresis and photopheresis instrument lines may be flushed with heparin as an anticoagulant and may pose a safety risk to patients with certain underlying conditions.

STANDARDS OF CARE

■ Caution should be exercised in apheresis and ECP procedures as the lines may be flushed with heparin, which may pose a risk to certain groups of patients. Consider using alternative anticoagulants such as citrate for such patients.

ERRORS INVOLVING SPECIFIC CLINICAL SCENARIOS

OCCULT ANEMIA—SEARCHING FOR A DELAYED HEMOLYTIC TRANSFUSION REACTION

Adverse reactions to transfused blood products range from innocuous mild allergic reactions to the transmission of incurable infections. The spectrum of symptoms for such transfusion reactions is broad, but it is most crucial to recognize and rule out an acute hemolytic reaction as this is one of the most likely sources for morbidity and mortality in transfusion medicine. The most severe and acute reactions stem from transfusion of ABO incompatible RBCs. Preformed, naturally occurring isohemagglutinins (anti-A and anti-B antibodies) can result in rapid and robust intravascular hemolysis. However, the effects of exposure to blood components may not be immediately apparent, but can be delayed for weeks, months, or longer.

Clinical Pitfall

Failure to recognize a clinically significant RBC antibody.

STANDARDS OF CARE

▦ In delayed transfusion reactions, the offending antibody can be found in the plasma, on the surface of the RBCs, or both. A DAT should be performed on all suspected cases. Acid elution studies can further help to identify a potentially anamnestic response.

IDENTIFICATION AND MANAGEMENT OF CLINICALLY SIGNIFICANT ALLOANTIBODIES IN PREGNANCY

HDFN is a disorder describing the immune-mediated destruction of fetal or neonatal RBCs. The clinical repercussions of HDFN have been substantially mitigated since the 1970s with the advent of routine postpartum prophylactic RhIG therapy. Yet despite reductions of approximately 90% in alloimmunization to RhD, continued clinical hemovigilance is necessary to prevent fetal and neonatal demise. Clinically significant alloantibodies, other than anti-D, can cross the placenta, resulting in RBC destruction. With ongoing loss of RBCs, the developing neonate will attempt to compensate physiologically by increasing the formation of immature RBCs (reticulocytosis). With the increased oxygen demand as a consequence of the loss of RBCs, the neonatal heart will be driven to compensate by increasing output—which can in turn lead to cardiac failure and fetal demise.

Clinical Pitfall

Failure to recognize clinically significant alloantibodies to minor RBC antigens that can cause severe HDFN.

STANDARDS OF CARE

- Fetal transfusion is most commonly performed using blood group O Rh-negative that is compatible with the implicated maternal antibody. These units should be leukoreduced, irradiated, and relatively fresh.
- Multiple transfusions can be performed to support the fetus through gestation to delivery. It is important to note that pregnant women receiving multiple transfusions secondary to HDFN often form multiple RBC antibodies.

LIBERAL VERSUS RESTRICTIVE TRANSFUSION STRATEGIES

Postsurgical anemia increases a patient's risk of death, particularly in the immediate postoperative setting and in the intensive care unit. The degree of asymptomatic anemia and subsequent decision to transfuse RBCs is a complex decision. Historical transfusion thresholds, coupled with nonevidence-based blood product ordering, have resulted in a renewed drive toward evidence-based decision making for RBC transfusions. The overall goal of RBC transfusion is to enhance tissue oxygenation, but the decision to transfuse must be balanced against other factors, such as potential risks of infection, alloimmunization, and general availability of the blood components.

Clinical Pitfall

Failure to follow evidence-based guidelines for managing asymptomatic anemia.

STANDARDS OF CARE

█ Studies from intensive care units have suggested a "trigger" for transfusion at an Hgb value of 7 g/dL. Controversy still remains regarding the effect of the age of the transfused RBC unit(s), with older units likely being inferior in quality (the "storage lesion" effect).

NONEVIDENCE-BASED PRACTICES IN PROPHYLACTIC PLATELET TRANSFUSIONS FOR MINOR PROCEDURES

Lumbar puncture (LP) is a common diagnostic and therapeutic procedure performed in both adult and pediatric patient populations. There is range of potential complications that can occur with LPs that includes headache, backache, cerebellar herniation, trauma to the conus medullaris, iatrogenic meningitis, and bleeding. Despite these complications, thrombocytopenia is by itself not a major contraindication to performing an LP on a patient. Nonetheless, the prophylactic platelet transfusion thresholds prior to performing an LP are controversial. Physicians performing this procedure are concerned about the risk for permanent neurologic injury.

Clinical Pitfall

Failure to recognize evidence-based platelet transfusion guidelines for minimally invasive procedures.

STANDARDS OF CARE

▨ Data to support a specific platelet count are limited. However, published reports on retrospective analyses and expert opinion support platelet counts greater than 10,000/μL to 50,000/μL. There are no data to support the need for a platelet count of 100,000/μL.

MOLECULAR DIFFERENCES IN THE RhD PROTEIN AND THE NEED FOR RhIG

The RhD protein is the most immunogenic of the Rh proteins. These proteins are expressed exclusively on the erythroid cells and can pose a significant risk for hemolytic transfusion reactions, as well as HDFN. The RhD protein is a transmembrane protein that has numerous variants based on alterations in the DNA sequence. Alterations in the DNA sequence often translate to structural changes in the RhD protein. Various mutations (deletion, single nucleotide polymorphism, and pseudogene) have been shown to alter different regions within the cytoplasmic, transmembrane, and external portion of the protein, each resulting in unique phenotypic protein expression.

If the protein alteration is on the external surface of the RBC, the changes in the three-dimensional structure of the protein are exposed to the immune system and can elicit different immune surveillance patterns. As a result, when patients with mutated extracellular branches of the RhD protein are transfused with RBCs from nonmutated donors, the recipient's immune system may recognize the external protein changes as foreign and mount an immune response. This structural alteration in the exposed extracellular part of the protein constitutes the biological basis for the immune response, termed "partial D." If the mutation in the RhD protein occurs on the intracellular portion of the protein, the resulting changes most frequently result in only a reduced level of expression of the RhD protein.

Clinical Pitfall

Failure to recognize the limitations of weak D/partial D antigen testing and their clinical significance.

STANDARDS OF CARE

- The first prenatal visit should include a thorough pregnancy history, as well as blood type and screen. At present, many FDA-approved reagents used for anti-D testing combine a monoclonal IgM antibody and a monoclonal or polyclonal IgG antibody, for the determination of a weak D.
- When the RhD typing of a patient is undertaken, a weak D test is not part of the standard of care. Only in situations where the infant of a mother is at risk for D alloimmunization will a weak D test be performed.

RECOGNITION OF IMMUNE-MEDIATED HEMOLYSIS IN A PEDIATRIC PATIENT

Approximately 20% of children in the United States will be anemic at some stage prior to their 18th birthday. The cause for this anemia is quite variable. Although immune hemolytic anemias more commonly affect adult populations, pediatric patients can also be affected. When present in pediatric populations the anemia frequently follows a postinfectious period. Immune-mediated anemias can be further classified, according to the implicated antibody-antigen reaction, as follows: warm autoimmune hemolytic anemia (WAIHA), CAD, mixed type autoimmune-mediated hemolytic anemia, drug-induced immune hemolytic anemia (DIIHA), and paroxysmal cold hemoglobinuria. Each of the disorders just named implicates an autoantibody directed against an RBC antigen that reduces the life span of the circulating RBC. The clinical severity of these disorders is variable and depends on the strength of the antibody–antigen interaction, the ability to fix complement on the RBC surface, and the range of temperatures at which the antibody is capable of binding to RBCs.

Clinical Pitfall

Failure to evaluate the patient for clinically significant immune-mediated hemolysis, resulting in delay of a correct diagnosis.

STANDARDS OF CARE

■ The Donath–Landsteiner test, an evaluation for a biphasic hemolysin, should be considered when a pediatric patient in the postinfectious period presents with a positive DAT with isolated complement fixation.

INAPPROPRIATE PLATELET TRANSFUSION FOR PATIENTS ON ASPIRIN

Platelet transfusions are critical interventions intended to aid in maintaining hemostasis. There are two licensed platelet products available in the United States: apheresis platelets and whole blood–derived platelet concentrates. Currently, the majority of platelet transfusions in the United States involves the use of apheresis platelet products (single donor) which, by AABB standards, should contain at least 3×10^{11} platelets in 90% of sampled units. Transfusion "triggers" or thresholds differ considerably depending on the clinical scenario and the patient's underlying disease. For example, in neurosurgical interventions, the consensus platelet threshold for the patient preoperatively is greater than $100,000/\mu L$.

Concomitant use of antiplatelet medications (eg, acetylsalicylic acid) can complicate the effectiveness of platelet transfusions. Aspirin irreversibly inhibits both cyclooxygenase-1 and 2 enzymes via acetylation. This irreversible inhibition prevents arachidonic acid conversion to thromboxane A2. The net effect of inhibiting thromboxane A2 generation is to reduce platelet aggregation.

Clinical Pitfall

Failure to consider aspirin pharmacology in platelet transfusion therapy.

STANDARDS OF CARE

- For neurosurgery, a consensus preprocedure platelet count is $100,000/\mu L$, although the optimal count remains to be determined.
- Rapid platelet function testing can be useful for optimizing platelet transfusions.

UNEXPECTED POSTTRANSFUSION PURPURA

The majority of platelet transfusions in the United States are administered prophylactically, secondary to thrombocytopenia. These transfusions are not devoid of risk and are susceptible to both infectious and noninfectious complications. Although acute reactions are more readily identified, delayed reactions to platelet transfusion can nonetheless cause significant morbidity and occasional mortality. Although rare, immunologic destruction of transfused platelets can occur. In pregnant patients, exposure to fetal platelet antigens can stimulate a maternal immune response leading to the severe clinical consequences of neonatal alloimmune thrombocytopenia (NAIT). Patients exposed to novel platelet antigens from platelet transfusions can also develop an immune response, causing a precipitous decrease in the platelet count that is usually only identified with serial measurements of the platelet count.

Clinical Pitfall

Failure to consider posttransfusion purpura (PTP) in the differential diagnosis of thrombocytopenia.

STANDARDS OF CARE

- PTP must be considered in the differential diagnosis of thrombocytopenia in patients exposed to platelet transfusions and in women who have been pregnant, particularly when the platelet count is very low.
- In cases of life-threatening bleeding, HPA-1a/1a negative units should be used for platelet transfusions unless platelet antigen testing suggests otherwise.

PHENOTYPE MATCHING TO MITIGATE ALLOIMMUNIZATION IN SICKLE CELL DISEASE

Worldwide, sickle cell disease (SCD) affects many different patient populations. In the United States, most cases of SCD affect African Americans. Despite multiple clinical trials demonstrating hydroxyurea as an effective therapy for acute life-threatening complications of SCD, RBC transfusion continues to be the more regularly performed therapy. Maintaining the Hgb S percentage below 30% during chronic transfusion therapy has been shown to reduce the risk of stroke.

The potential for increased alloimmunization and consequent hemolytic transfusion reactions is increased by the high degree of variability in antigen matching between the recipient and donor blood products. It is known that the rate of alloimmunization in patients with SCD is disproportionately higher than in other chronically transfused patient populations. The etiology of this discrepancy is not fully understood.

Clinical Pitfall

Failure to recognize the potential risk of alloimmunization in a chronically transfused patient.

STANDARDS OF CARE

▓ For patients requiring chronic transfusion support (eg, SCD, thalassemia, and other hemoglobinopathies), there is currently no universal standard; however, studies have demonstrated that prophylactic phenotype matching for the RhCE and K antigens results in reduction in alloimmunization rates to minor RBC antigens.

REFUSING BLOOD TRANSFUSION: WHEN PATIENT AND PHYSICIAN BELIEFS FAIL TO ALIGN

The medical and surgical management of patients who refuse allogeneic and/or autologous blood is complex. The genesis of such decisions can be religious, cultural, and/or personal in nature, and is not limited to patients who identify themselves as Jehovah's Witness. The refusal of blood transfusion may conflict with the medical responsibility for preserving life, yet the decision by a competent and informed adult patient to decline treatment must be respected, even if there are clear medical indications for such a transfusion.

Clinical Pitfall

Failure to respect and understand the patient's autonomy regarding their care.

STANDARDS OF CARE

▓ A competent adult has the legal right to make decisions about receiving a blood transfusion. In the event of a life-threatening blood loss, a court order is not required for transfusion of a recipient who is a minor (even if the legal guardian says no).

CRYPT ANTIGEN ACTIVATION, ADVERSE CONSEQUENCES

T activation, also known as the Thomsen–Hubener–Friedenrich phenomenon, is an enzymatic modification of the RBC membrane proteins that exposes, or "activates," the normally "cryptic" (hidden) T, or Thomsen, antigen. The T antigen is normally sequestered on cellular membranes until it is exposed through the removal of N-acetyl-neuraminic acid (sialic acid) residues by neuraminidase, an enzyme produced by a variety of organisms such as Clostridia and *Streptococcus pneumoniae*. Adult plasma contains naturally preformed antibodies to crypt antigens. Such transfused plasma can thus propagate an ongoing immune-mediated hemolysis.

Clinical Pitfall

Failure to consider cryptic antigen exposure and to understand the associated transfusion risks.

STANDARDS OF CARE

▨ Washing of blood products may be necessary to reduce the risk of passive anti-T transmission.
▨ Consideration of crypt antigen exposure in patients with infections should be factored into decisions.

FAILURE TO RECOGNIZE SPECIFIC RISK FACTORS THAT ARE ASSOCIATED WITH ADVERSE REACTIONS IN BLOOD DONORS

Healthy persons can donate up to 500 mL of blood with only a transient impact on their circulatory system (the

FDA limits donation to 10.5 mL/kg). Nonetheless, syncopal episodes do occur among blood donors. The incidence ranges between 2% and 5% of all donors, and is especially common in first time donors mostly due to anxiety and vasovagal reactions.

Clinical Pitfall

Failure to recognize risk factors for syncopal reactions in blood donors.

STANDARDS OF CARE

■ Young age, gender, first time donation, and anxiety are known risk factors for postdonation syncope. Donors who meet these criteria should be carefully monitored.

MISINTERPRETATION OF THE DAT

The DAT, also known as the direct antiglobulin or Coombs' test, indicates whether antibody (IgG) and/or complement (usually C3d) is bound to the patient's RBCs. A positive DAT can have various interpretations and requires appropriate additional testing. The DAT should be interpreted in the context of the patient's medical history and underlying condition. Thus, the clinical significance of a positive DAT should be determined by taking account of both clinical and laboratory information.

A positive DAT can be succeeded by an elution assay in which antibody adhering to the patient's RBCs is removed from these cells and evaluated, with the goal of determining whether alloantibodies not detected in the patient's plasma are adhering to the RBCs. The eluted antibody can either be identical to that found in the plasma or may represent an additional underlying alloantibody not detected in the plasma. How such antibody elutions are performed also depends on whether the patient has been recently transfused. A positive DAT is often misinterpreted as being indicative of RBC hemolysis, but caution should be exercised as there are other causes of a positive DAT.

Clinical Pitfall

Failure to understand multiple causes of a positive DAT.

STANDARDS OF CARE

- A positive DAT should be interpreted in the context of the underlying disease and results of the associated laboratory tests. It may be clinically insignificant or may be associated with an underlying disease, such as autoimmune hemolytic anemia (AIHA), drug-induced anemia, or HDFN.
- In the setting of antibody identification, performing an eluate in which antibodies are removed from the patient's RBCs for further testing may sometimes be useful as it very occasionally reveals the presence of an alloantibody not present in the plasma.
- In the setting of a transfusion reaction, a DAT should be performed on posttransfusion as well as on the pretransfusion samples of the blood, in order to determine whether the strength of the reaction has increased. Especially if the DAT has increased in strength, an eluate should be performed to determine the specificity of the antibody coating the RBCs.

WARFARIN REVERSAL—INAPPROPRIATE USE OF FFP

Warfarin (Coumadin) exerts its anticoagulant effect by inhibiting the hepatic synthesis of the clotting factors II, VII, IX, and X (as well as protein C and protein S). All these factors depend on the active form of vitamin K for synthesis. Vitamin K administration usually corrects the anticoagulant effect of warfarin, but the time required for correction depends on the dose of vitamin K and on the route of vitamin K administration (IV is fastest; oral is slowest). In nonemergent situations when the bleeding is not significant, withholding the warfarin and administering vitamin K are sufficient. With significant bleeding or if emergent surgery is required, plasma or prothrombin complex concentrates (PCCs) are also usually administered. Four-factor PCC preparations that include factor VII can more immediately reverse the warfarin effect, but these PCCs are as yet not available in the United States, despite being well tolerated in patients. PCCs can also be administered more quickly and in smaller volumes and on that basis are advantageous for emergent reversal of warfarin.

In anticoagulant-associated intracerebral hemorrhage (AAICH) that occurs with significant bleeding, vitamin K should be immediately administered to the patient. It is usually given together with FFP or PCCs because vitamin K depends on hepatic synthesis of new coagulation factors and takes hours to induce coagulation factor synthesis. The intravenous route for vitamin K may be preferred as this works faster than oral or subcutaneous routes.

Although FFP may be readily available and contains all the coagulation factors, administration is relatively slow and replacement of factors may still be insufficient. Administering FFP alone is not appropriate in AAICH with concomitant bleeding, not only because administration is relatively slow but also because the larger volumes required to achieve the desired effect may not be tolerated by the patient.

Recombinant factor VIIa (rFVIIa) promptly reverses a prolonged INR in warfarin users, but it does not substitute for all four of the decreased clotting factors; it is generally not recommended for warfarin reversal.

Clinical Pitfall

Failure to recognize that warfarin reversal for severe bleeding requires treatment with vitamin K as well as with FFP.

STANDARDS OF CARE

■ Several differing international guidelines are available for warfarin reversal in the context of intracerebral hemorrhage, most of which recommend intravenous vitamin K supplemented with either FFP or PCCs, as vitamin K alone is not considered adequate.

■ In settings that do not involve significant bleeding, the 2012 CHEST guidelines recommend achieving anticoagulation broadly as follows:

   i. Patients taking vitamin K antagonists and with INRs between 4.5 and 10, but with no evidence of bleeding, do not need to routinely take vitamin K.

   ii. Patients with INRs greater than 10, with no evidence of bleeding, should take oral vitamin K.

■ In cases of serious bleeding in patients with warfarin-associated ICH, recent guidelines recommend a vitamin K dose of 10 mg given intravenously at a slow infusion rate (over 30 minutes) with consideration of a repeat dose at 12 hours. Supplementation with either FFP, PCCs, or factor VIIa is generally considered necessary for rapid correction of the INR, but evidence-based guidance and correlated outcomes for each of these therapies is lacking.

■ The use of plasma in the setting of warfarin-induced ICH was recently given only a "weak" recommendation by the AABB. This low grading may be due to delayed administration and inadequate dosing of the product. A minimum of 15 mL/kg and ≤30 mL/kg has been recommended, unless the patient cannot tolerate the volume.

■ Four-factor PCCs are effective for patients with AAICH, whereas the benefit of three-factor PCC therapy has not been fully established and is therefore as yet not approved for AAICH. Recent randomized clinical trials showed that four-factor PCCs had a similar hemostatic efficacy to plasma at 24 hours in patients requiring warfarin reversal and were actually superior to plasma in achieving target INR correction within 30 minutes after infusion.

■ The American Heart Association and American Stroke Association do not recommend the routine use of factor VIIa for warfarin reversal for AAICH.

ANTI-KELL ALLOANTIBODIES—MISSED DIAGNOSIS OF HDFN

HDFN occurs mostly through maternal alloimmunization against an antigen present on fetal RBCs (more rarely, it can also occur through prior maternal transfusion). The maternal antibody crosses the placenta and coats the fetal RBCs, which are then removed from circulation by splenic macrophages, resulting in fetal anemia. The titer of the maternal alloantibody can be helpful in monitoring the potential for HDFN. Amniotic fluid bilirubin levels can also serve as an indicator of active hemolysis. Both of these results should, however, be interpreted with caution when anti-Kell alloantibodies are implicated in the disorder. Newer approaches to diagnosing HDFN use Doppler measurements of peak systolic blood flow velocity in the fetal middle cerebral artery (MCA).

Clinical Pitfall

Failure to understand the role in HDFN of maternal antibodies that suppress erythropoiesis and cause anemia without causing hemolysis.

STANDARDS OF CARE

■ After the risk of HDFN has been established through prenatal and neonatal testing for maternal alloimmunization as well as phenotyping of the biological father's RBCs (and fetal phenotyping or genotyping to determine the antigen status of the fetus), maternal antibody titers to the implicated antigen should be measured every two to four weeks, beginning at 18 weeks gestational age.

▪ Amniotic fluid bilirubin levels can be helpful for monitoring hemolysis but should be interpreted with caution when anti-Kell group antibodies are implicated, as fetal anemia may be driven by suppression of erythropoiesis rather than by active RBC hemolysis.

IgA DEFICIENCY—MISINTERPRETATIONS AND ASSUMPTIONS

IgA deficiency is relatively common: about 1 in 900 in donors of European descent in the United States and United Kingdom, but about 1:500 in Finland; and only about 1:18,500 in Japan. However, only 20% to 30% of IgA deficient individuals will form an anti-IgA antibody (80% in individuals with autoimmune disease). If IgA deficiency is suspected, an IgA level should be ordered. If IgA is severely deficient (<0.05 mg/dL), the presence of an anti-IgA antibody should be determined. A search for IgA deficient donors should be initiated, as finding such donors can take time. Some tests for IgA involve nephelometry, which is usually not sufficiently sensitive to identify the level of severity of deficiency associated with the production of an anti-IgA antibody.

Anti-IgA may be present as a natural autoantibody detected in normal human sera, and/or as an alloantibody. It can be stimulated by exposure to IgA, but is also formed regardless of previous transfusion or pregnancy. Anti-IgA is usually of the IgG class, but it can also be IgE or IgM and can be of variable specificity. Not all individuals with IgA deficiency and anti-IgA antibody will have anaphylactic reactions. Conversely, it is also important to note that anaphylactic reactions have been noted in IgA deficient patients who have no detectable anti-IgA antibody.

Severe allergic/anaphylactic reactions require immediate discontinuation of the transfusion, with maintenance of open intravenous line access, the availability of oxygen (sometimes requiring intubation), and usually treatment with epinephrine (as well as possibly vasopressors, steroids, and/or H1 and H2 receptor antagonists). Common symptoms seen in anaphylaxis include dyspnea, laryngeal edema, circulatory collapse, and hypotension. Fever is usually absent.

Clinical Pitfall

Failure to appropriately follow up a presumed diagnosis of IgA deficiency.

STANDARDS OF CARE

When an anaphylactic transfusion reaction occurs and IgA deficiency is suspected:

- If IgA deficiency is less than 0.05 mg/dL, check for the presence IgA antibody.
- Initiate search for blood products from IgA deficient patients.
- If IgA deficient products are not available, give washed RBCs and washed platelet products.
- Plasma and cryoprecipitate for IgA deficient patients must be collected from IgA deficient donors.
- Premedication with steroids and antihistamines may be beneficial.
- Do not assume that the absence of an anti-IgA antibody precludes anaphylaxis due to IgA deficiency, or conversely that individuals with IgA deficiency and an anti-IgA antibody will necessarily have anaphylactic reactions.

MISINTERPRETING THE CAUSE OF HYPOTENSION DURING TRANSFUSION

The differential diagnosis for hypotension associated with transfusion includes acute hemolytic reactions, anaphylaxis, and bacterial contamination with sepsis. Hypotension associated with sepsis is usually accompanied with a fever greater than 38.5°C, rigors, and vomiting during transfusion, often with the added complications of shock, oliguria, and disseminated intravascular coagulation. As with all suspected transfusion reactions, the first step is to stop the transfusion while maintaining an open intravenous access line. Severe allergic/anaphylactic reactions require immediate discontinuation of the transfusion, with appropriate supportive treatment to maintain oxygenation and blood pressure. However, hypotension may also be unrelated to the transfusion and instead be due to the patient's underlying condition.

By definition, a primary hypotensive transfusion reaction occurs as an isolated decrease in systolic and/or diastolic blood pressure of 30 mmHg or more within minutes of starting transfusion and resolves with supportive treatment soon after the transfusion is stopped. Such hypotensive reactions may be due to blood passing through charged filters (usually negatively charged) in patients who are taking angiotensin-converting enzyme inhibitors (ACE-i). In such patients on ACE-i receiving blood through negatively charged filters, the generation of bradykinin and/or its metabolite *des-Arg-bradykinin* appear to be implicated.

Clinical Pitfall

Failure to fully explore the potential causes for hypotension in a patient being transfused.

STANDARDS OF CARE

- Hypotension in the setting of a transfusion should be carefully evaluated and not assumed to be due to the patient's underlying condition. Each option in the differential diagnosis should be considered in the context of the patient's past medical history, clinical scenario, and the laboratory results.

▓ Knowing a patient's medications is important in analyzing a suspected transfusion reaction. In patients undergoing total plasma exchange (TPE), ACE-i can interact with charged membrane surfaces in the apheresis instrument. These drugs should therefore be discontinued prior to starting TPE (at least 24 hours before starting apheresis in patients on short-acting ACE-i such as captopril and quinapril; or several days before starting apheresis in the case of longer acting ACE inhibitors such as enalapril and lisinopril).

▓ If the hypotension is accompanied by significant fever, bacterial contamination should be ruled out by culturing the blood product.

INAPPROPRIATE APPLICATION OF PREMEDICATION FOR TRANSFUSION

Allergic and febrile nonhemolytic transfusion reactions (FNHTRs) are the most commonly reported transfusion reactions. They are generally mild and do not cause significant morbidity. FNHTRs are isolated febrile reactions that occur during transfusions that are not associated with any hemolysis. Mild allergic reactions can be treated by temporarily stopping the transfusion and administering diphenhydramine, and resuming transfusion if the patient is stable. Such isolated reactions generally do not necessitate routine premedication for subsequent transfusions.

Acetaminophen and diphenhydramine are generally considered effective therapies for fever and allergy, respectively. In the setting of transfusion, however, their routine usage is controversial since their efficacy has not been proven, and because fever and allergic reactions from transfusion are often temporally limited and self-resolving. Nonetheless, it is estimated that physicians routinely prescribe these medications in up to 80% of blood product transfusions in order to avert the possibility of reactions. In some institutions, all transfusions receive premedication.

The tendency to premedicate is usually greater if the patient has previously suffered an allergic or febrile reaction while undergoing transfusion. The medical record is not always reviewed to determine if there was ever an indication for such medication. Patients who have experienced an isolated allergic or febrile reaction associated with transfusion are most often no more likely to have a repeat reaction than those who have never experienced a reaction.

Acetaminophen and diphenhydramine are both associated with potential toxicities and should not be routinely, and without good reason, administered to patients prior to transfusion. For severe transfusion reactions, more effective alternatives to these medications are also available.

Clinical Pitfall

Failure to recognize that universal routine premedication with diphenhydramine and acetaminophen does not prevent or reduce the rate of allergic and/or FNHTR transfusion reactions.

STANDARDS OF CARE

- Mild allergic reactions, such as hives, associated with transfusion can be treated by temporarily stopping the transfusion, maintaining open intravenous access, and waiting for the symptoms to subside before resuming transfusion at a slower rate under close observation and monitoring.
- Diphenhydramine (or other antihistamines) can be judiciously used to treat an urticarial reaction but should not be routinely given as a prophylactic premedication.
- For recurring and severe reactions, alternatives to premedication such as washed or plasma-reduced products may be helpful. For severe allergic reactions,

alternative medications such as antihistamines other than diphenhydramine, H1 receptor antagonists, and corticosteroids may be helpful, but their efficacy has not been unequivocally established.

INCOMPLETE EVALUATION OF PLATELET REFRACTORINESS

Thrombocytopenia is associated with a broad range of medical conditions. The causes of refractory thrombocytopenia (when the count does not increase despite transfusion of platelets) are both immune and nonimmune, and often multifactorial. Treatment of the underlying illness will frequently alleviate nonimmune causes of refractoriness. Immune-mediated causes may require HLA-matched or crossmatched platelets.

To distinguish immune from nonimmune cases of refractory thrombocytopenia, it is essential that the peripheral blood platelet count be performed accurately. For an increment in the platelet count to be accurate, it should be measured between 15 and 60 minutes immediately following completion of the platelet transfusion. The increment in the count should be determined using the corrected count increment (CCI—see Standards of Care) that takes into account the patient's size via a body surface area measurement. Obese patients with large blood volumes and patients with splenomegaly who have sequestration of platelets from circulation may show peripheral blood platelet counts that are corrected by the calculation of the CCI. The CCI should be calculated following two consecutive platelet transfusions before making a determination of "platelet refractoriness."

Since the introduction and widespread implementation of uniform prestorage leukoreduction, the immune causes of platelet refractoriness via alloimmunization to HLA Class 1 antigens have decreased. Platelets express HLA Class IA and IB antigens.

Matched platelets can be selected either by HLA antigen-based selection, or by crossmatching which does not require knowledge of HLA type.

An unreliable platelet count increment following transfusion may lead to either the unnecessary transfusion of additional platelets to increase the count or to a premature determination of "refractoriness."

Clinical Pitfall

Failure to take a platelet count between 15 and 60 minutes following transfusion and to calculate the CCI before making a determination of platelet refractoriness.

STANDARDS OF CARE

▦ Determine the platelet count within 15 to 60 minutes following transfusion of platelets.

▦ From the platelet count, calculate the CCI, taking into account the patient's specific body surface area, using the formula:

$$CCI = \frac{Body\ surface\ area\,(m^2) \times Platelet\ count\ increment\,(platelets\,/\,\mu L) \times 10^{11}}{Number\ of\ platelets\ transfused}$$

▦ Perform two consecutive platelet counts and CCI calculations before making a determination of "platelet refractoriness."

▦ Rule out nonimmune causes of refractoriness before ordering HLA-matched platelets to manage alloimmunization to HLA class I antigens.

THROMBOTIC THROMBOCYTOPENIC PURPURA—MISSED DIAGNOSIS

TTP is classically diagnosed by the "pentad" of anemia, thrombocytopenia, neurologic signs, fever, and renal failure. While the ADAMTS13 assay can yield a more rapid and potentially accurate measurement of the disease, its utility in acute management of TTP is disputable. The full pentad of symptoms is not always observed in patients presenting with TTP. While fever is present in 24% of patients, neurologic signs in 63%, and renal abnormalities in 60%, each of the conditions can also manifest in a variety of ways; and nonspecific symptoms such as nausea, weakness, and abdominal pain may further confuse the diagnosis. More importantly, the absence of fever, neurologic signs, or renal dysfunction does not preclude a diagnosis of TTP.

The diagnosis of TTP should be seriously considered in patients with thrombocytopenia and microangiopathic hemolytic anemia (MAHA) presenting in the absence of an underlying disease. MAHA is diagnosed in the setting of a hemolytic anemia by the simultaneous presence, on a peripheral blood smear, of schistocytes. The diagnosis of hemolytic anemia is further suggested by elevated values for serum LDH, indirect bilirubin, and reticulocyte count.

As MAHA and thrombocytopenia are not specific for TTP, other causes for these conditions should also be evaluated through additional laboratory tests, such as the PT, PTT, a DAT, and liver function tests. In short, the diagnosis of TTP should not be too strictly based on the recognition of the classic pentad.

Clinical Pitfall

Failure to correctly diagnose TTP.

STANDARDS OF CARE

- The diagnosis of TTP can be made based on unexplained MAHA and thrombocytopenia and does not require the classic "pentad" of symptoms that includes fever, neurologic symptoms, and renal dysfunction.
- TPE is typically performed for one TPE daily until the platelet count is above 150,000/μL, and is then often continued for two more days after this platelet count is achieved.

■ Blood samples for laboratory tests such as ADAMTS13 should be collected before commencing plasma exchanges or transfusions, and caution should be used in the interpretation of ADAMTS13 values.

TRANSFUSION-RELATED ACUTE LUNG INJURY—FAILURE TO DIAGNOSE

The diagnosis of transfusion-related acute lung injury (TRALI) is based on a set of consensus criteria that involves both clinical and radiologic findings. These criteria serve as a guide only, and a high level of suspicion should be maintained for diagnosing this disease given its relatively high (transfusion related) mortality. Respiratory distress in the absence of left atrial hypertension (circulatory overload) occurring within 6 hours of transfusion should alert the physician to the possibility of TRALI. Patients with TRALI also do not, by the consensus criteria, have pretransfusion lung injury. However, mild and atypical cases presenting with symptoms such as only mild shortness of breath should not preclude consideration of a possible diagnosis of TRALI, even though the symptoms may not completely fit the consensus criteria.

The exact pathogenesis of TRALI is unknown but usually involves anti-HLA antibodies (and/or antineutrophil antibodies) that trigger a cascade of events resulting in bilateral lung infiltrates involving both interstitial and alveolar spaces. In some cases, the presentation of TRALI following RBC transfusions is thought to be mediated by RBC membrane components, specifically lysophosphatidylcholine.

The presence of the pathogenic antibodies can be determined with tests such as the panel reactive antibody (PRA) assay although this assay will not detect antineutrophil antibodies or biologically activated lipids that can also cause TRALI.

Clinical Pitfall

Failure to consider a diagnosis of TRALI when the presenting symptoms are mild or atypical.

STANDARDS OF CARE

▨ Given the relative mortality risk of TRALI, a high index of suspicion should be maintained even when symptoms are mild, especially in the setting of other possible disease etiologies. The Canadian Consensus Panel and the NIH criteria for TRALI should generally be applied in diagnosing the condition, but a high level of suspicion should nonetheless be maintained for mild and atypical cases.

▨ Plasma units from donors (especially female; multiparous) should be analyzed for anti-HLA Class I or Class II antibodies (or antineutrophil antibodies). When such antibodies are discovered, the patient is typically tested for the cognate antigen to understand whether an antibody–antigen interaction may have triggered the transfusion reaction. Donors of positive units should be excluded from further donation of plasma, but they may be allowed to donate platelets.

FAILURE TO RECOGNIZE THAT SERIOUS, POTENTIALLY FATAL HEMOLYTIC TRANSFUSION REACTIONS CAN OCCUR WITH BLOOD PRODUCTS

Severe allergic reactions can occur in response to plasma proteins or other agents contained in blood products. Type I hypersensitivity responses occur very rapidly following contact with the relevant antigens and recur on subsequent occasions via an IgE-mediated degranulation of mast cells and basophils. The organ systems affected include skin and the mucosa of the gastrointestinal and respiratory tracts, where vascular leakage and tissue edema may occur. Arterial dilatation may cause headache and hypotension, whereas bronchoconstriction can cause respiratory distress. The mediators of these responses include histamine, serotonin and bradykinin, lymphokines, leukotrienes, and the anaphylatoxins C3a and C5a.

Clinical Pitfall

Failure to be prepared for anaphylactic transfusion reactions, particularly following rapid platelet transfusions.

STANDARDS OF CARE

- Supportive care (Advanced Cardiac Life Support and ICU support) should be readily available.
- Platelets should be transfused slowly and by gravity. Although platelets can be given via a pump, they should never be given by rapid infusion.
- IgA deficient patients, especially those with documented anaphylactic reactions, should be transfused with products derived from other IgA-deficient blood donors or with washed cellular blood products.

FAILURE TO RECOGNIZE DRUG-INDUCED HEMOLYTIC ANEMIA

Drug-induced hemolytic anemia (DIHA) is a rare complication occurring in less than one in a million individuals. Drugs may induce the generation of an antibody against RBCs that recognize the RBC only in the presence of the drug (classic form). However, they may also generate true autoantibodies to RBCs that do not require the presence of the drug for recognition. The number of drugs now known to be associated with DIHA is about 130. The most frequently implicated drugs are piperacillin and the cephalosporins.

At least four explanatory mechanisms of DIHA have been described. One such mechanism entails binding of the drug to the RBC membrane, which then elicits an antibody directed largely to the drug itself that can lead to extravascular hemolysis.

Clinical Pitfall

Failure to diagnose DIHA in a critically ill patient receiving medications known to be implicated in the disease.

STANDARDS OF CARE

▓ DIHA should be considered in patients who present with unexplained anemia, particularly if they are receiving drugs associated with DIHA.

FAILURE TO RECOGNIZE THAT DONOR HIV EXPOSURE IS ASSOCIATED WITH A SPECIFIC FEDERALLY MANDATED PROCESS FOR RECIPIENT NOTIFICATION

A look-back investigation on the transfusion service identifies potential transfusion-infected recipients and the implicated donors. For some disease entities, such as HIV, federal regulations guide the investigations. Transmission of HIV through transfusion of contaminated blood components was documented in the United States in 1982. Virtually all of these transfusion-associated cases occurred before 1985, when HIV antibody testing was not available. Since then, the risk for transfusion-transmitted HIV infection has been almost eliminated through the use of questionnaires to exclude the high risk donor, and through the application of sensitive laboratory screening tests to identify infected blood donors.

The risk for acquiring HIV infection through blood transfusion today is estimated conservatively to be about one in two million, based on 2007 to 2008 data.

When a blood collection center identifies a donor whose blood may be infected with hepatitis C virus (HCV), HIV-1, and/or HIV-2, written notification of the infection is sent to all medical directors of blood banks that might have received previous blood products from that infected donor. Federal regulations also contain stipulations regarding such notifications about infected donors.

Clinical Pitfall

Failure to be informed of the FDA-mandated regulations governing donor and recipient notifications about HIV and/or HCV infected blood products.

STANDARDS OF CARE

- Consent must be obtained from all patients for blood product administration. As part of that consent process, the risk of infectious diseases, including HIV and HCV, must be addressed. The physician and blood bank should keep a record of these notifications and test results.
- When supplemental testing for HIV or HCV is positive, the transfusion service medical director is responsible for notifying the donor as well as all patients who may be affected.
- Reasonable attempts must be made to notify the recipient within eight weeks after receiving the donor testing results.
- A legal representative or relative of the recipient should be notified if the recipient is a minor, deceased, or adjudged incompetent.
- At least three attempts to notify the affected parties must be made.

RISK OF HYPERKALEMIA FROM RBC TRANSFUSION

Damage to the red cell membrane or lysis of the RBC results in release of intracellular potassium.

Complications of hyperkalemia can arise in patients after receiving multiple RBC transfusions. A major determinant of the risk of hyperkalemia following transfusion is the potassium concentration of the unit. However, other factors are also involved, including the age of the patient, presence of tissue hypoperfusion, and the effects on the patient of the rate of transfusion. Pediatric patients with cardiac disease are particularly sensitive to hyperkalemia. Many institutions wash RBCs to reduce total potassium load prior to issuing units to pediatric cardiac surgery patients. However, adults with poor cardiac output are also at risk.

Clinical Pitfall

Failure to recognize that hyperkalemia may be associated with RBC transfusions.

STANDARDS OF CARE

- Irradiated RBC units should ideally be used within 6 to 8 hours of irradiation, although AABB standards allow longer out-dates.
- If issue of irradiated products within 6 to 8 hours is not possible, efforts should nonetheless be made not to issue these units to the surgical or ICU patient populations, as they are at higher risk for the metabolic derangements associated with hyperkalemic cardiac complications.

FAILURE TO RECOGNIZE THAT INTENSIVE PLASMA EXCHANGE CAN CAUSE METABOLIC ALKALOSIS

TTP is a rare blood condition that causes microthrombi to form in small blood vessels throughout the body. Classically, the following five features are indicative of TTP: neurologic symptoms, kidney failure, fever, thrombocytopenia, and MAHA. For unclear reasons, the kidney microvasculature is particularly sensitive to the formation of microthrombi, and some level of kidney dysfunction is, therefore, present in many TTP patients. TPE with donor plasma as fluid replacement is the first-line therapy for TTP, a life-threatening disease with considerable mortality (despite the efficacy of TPE). TPE is typically performed daily until the platelet count and LDH are back in the normal range.

Clinical Pitfall

Failure to correctly assess the source of metabolic alkalosis resulting from blood products during intensive TPE.

STANDARDS OF CARE

■ Patients receiving large amounts of plasma, particularly those with renal insufficiency, should be assessed with venous pH and bicarbonate measurements because of the risk of metabolic alkalosis.

FAILURE TO RECOGNIZE THE RISK OF ALLOIMMUNE THROMBOCYTOPENIA IN A PRIMIGRAVIDA

NAIT occurs as a result of maternal alloimmunization to fetal platelet antigens that lead to the destruction of fetal platelets. Unlike HDFN, in which fetal anemia develops due to maternal sensitization of fetal red cell antigens and hemolysis arises in second or later pregnancies, one third to one half of infants with NAIT are affected during the first pregnancy. The mechanism of cellular destruction is analogous to that of red cell incompatibility and destruction that occurs in HDFN.

Transplacental passage of fetal platelets in early second trimester sensitizes the mother, who produces IgG antibodies directed against platelet specific (or more rarely HLA) antigens of paternal origin on the fetal platelets. The neonate may present with a bleeding diathesis of variable severity after birth, or more rarely in utero. NAIT complicates 1.5 per 1,000 to 1 per 5,000 live birth Caucasian births. Although NAIT accounts for only 3% of all general fetal and neonatal thrombocytopenias (<150,000/µL), it accounts for about 30% of all severe thrombocytopenias with platelet counts of less than 50,000/µL.

Clinical Pitfall

Failure to understand that passive alloimmune destruction of platelets in neonates can occur in first pregnancies.

STANDARDS OF CARE

- NAIT should be considered in the differential diagnosis of newborns with thrombocytopenia, even for first pregnancies. Laboratory testing should be used to determine the specificity of the implicated antigen/antibody.
- Prophylactic transfusions are often recommended for low-neonatal platelet counts ranging between 30,000 and 50,000/µL.
- After a first case of NAIT, subsequent pregnancies should be carefully monitored for the development of NAIT. The mother can also receive prenatal treatment with IVIG.

UNNECESSARY PLATELET TRANSFUSIONS

The causal relationship between thrombocytopenia and an increased risk of bleeding is well established. Recommendations for a threshold number of platelets to prompt transfusion for in-patients, without any clinical bleeding, range between 5,000 and 10,000/µL. In the treatment of leukemias, only limited guidance is available on prophylactic platelet transfusion triggers for minor procedures such as central venous line placement.

Clinical Pitfall

Failure to recognize the appropriate prophylactic trigger for transfusion of platelets.

STANDARDS OF CARE

- A generally accepted platelet transfusion threshold for a "nonbleeding" in-hospital patient, without any coagulopathy, is 10,000/μL.
- Current recommendations for platelet transfusion thresholds for surgeries are 50,000/μL. The response to a platelet transfusion is best assessed by obtaining a posttransfusion platelet count. This should be obtained between 15 and 60 minutes after completion of the transfusion. The effectiveness of the response is assessed by calculating a CCI (see case "Incomplete Evaluation of Platelet Refractoriness" on page 39).

BIBLIOGRAPHY

Amrein K, Schmid P, Mansouri Taleghani B. Delayed haemolytic transfusion reaction initially presenting as serum sickness like syndrome. *Eur J Intern Med.* 2009;20:e122–e123.

Ansell J, Hirsh J, Hylek E, et al. Pharmacology and management of the vitamin K antagonists. *Chest.* 2008;133(suppl):160S–198S.

Bamberger DH. Mercy Hospital, Inc. v. Jackson: a recurring dilemma for health care providers in the treatment of Jehovah's Witnesses. *MD Law Rev.* 1987;46:514–532.

Bassler D, Greinacher A, Okascharoen C, et al. A systematic review and survey of the management of unexpected neonatal alloimmune thrombocytopenia. *Transfusion.* 2008;48:92–98.

Berentsen S, Beiske K, Tjønnfjord GE. Primary chronic cold agglutinin disease: an update on pathogenesis, clinical features and therapy. *Hematology.* 2007;12(5):361–370.

Berry-Dortch S, Woodside CH, Boral LI. Limitations of the immediate spin crossmatch when used for detecting ABO incompatibility. *Transfusion.* 1985;25:176–178.

Bessos H, Seghatchian J. What's happening? The expanding role of apheresis platelet support in neonatal alloimmune thrombocytopenia: current status and future trends. *Transfus Apher Sci.* 2005;33:191–197.

Billote DB, Glisson SN, Green D, Wixson RL. A prospective, randomized study of preoperative autologous blood donation for hip replacement surgery. *J Bone Joint Surg Am.* 2002;84-A:1299–1304.

Brecher ME, Goodnough LT. The rise and fall of preoperative autologous blood donation. *Transfusion.* 2002;42:1618–1622.

Broderick JP, Brott TG, Duldner JE, et al. Volume of intracerebral hemorrhage. A powerful and easy-to-use predictor of 30-day mortality. *Stroke.* 1993;24:987–993.

Brott T, Broderick J, Kothari R, et al. Early hemorrhage growth in patients with intracerebral hemorrhage. *Stroke.* 1997;28:1–5.

Buchta C, Felfernig M, Höcker P, et al. Stability of coagulation factors in thawed, solvent/detergent-treated plasma during storage at 4 degrees C for 6 days. *Vox Sang.* 2004;87:182–186.

Carson JL, Duff A, Poses RM, et al. Effect of anaemia and cardiovascular disease on surgical mortality and morbidity. *Lancet.* 1996;348:1055–1060.

Centers for Disease Control and Prevention (CDC). HIV transmission through transfusion—Missouri and Colorado, 2008. *MMWR Morb Mortal Wkly Rep.* 2010;59(41): 1335–1339.

Chowdary P, Saayman AG, Paulus U, et al. Efficacy of standard dosing and 30 mL/kg fresh frozen plasma in correcting laboratory parameters of haemostasis in critically ill patients. *Br J Haematol.* 2004;125:69–73.

Copelovitch L, Kaplan BS. Streptococcus pneumonia-associated hemolytic uremic syndrome: classification and the emergence of serotype 19A. *Pediatrics.* 2010;125:e174–e182.

Coppo P, Wolf M, Veyradier A, et al. Prognostic value of inhibitory anti-ADAMTS13 antibodies in adult-acquired thrombotic thrombocytopenic purpura. *Br J Haematol.* 2006;132:66–74.

Costanzo MR, Dipchand A, Starling R, et al. The International Society of Heart and Lung Transplantation guidelines for the care of heart transplant recipients. *J Heart Lung Transplant.* 2010;29:914–956.

Crookston KP, Reiner AP, Cooper LJ, et al. RBC T activation and hemolysis: implications for pediatric transfusion management. *Transfusion.* 2000;40:801–812.

Das SS, Chaudhary R, Khetan D. A comparison of conventional tube test and gel technique in evaluation of direct antiglobulin test. *Hematology.* 2007;12:175–178.

Davis A, Mandal R, Johnson M, et al. A touch of TRALI. *Transfusion.* 2008;48:541–545.

Denomme GA, Wagner FF, Fernandes BJ, et al. Partial D, weak D types, and novel RHD alleles among 33,864 multiethnic patients: implications for anti-D alloimmunization and prevention. *Transfusion.* 2005;45:1554–1560.

Duran JA, González AA, García DD, et al. Best blood sample draw site during liver transplantation. *Transplant Proc.* 2009;41(3):991–993.

Dzik S. How I do it: platelet support for refractory patients. *Transfusion.* 2007;47:374–378.

Eder AF. Update on HDFN: new information on long-standing controversies. *Immunohematology.* 2006;22: 188–195.

Eder AF, Hillyer CD, Dy BA, et al. Adverse reactions to allogeneic whole blood donation by 16- and 17-year-olds. *JAMA.* 2008;299:2279–2286.

Eder AF, Manno CS. Does red-cell T activation matter? *Br J Hematol.* 2001;114:25–30.

Flaherty ML. Anticoagulant-associated intracerebral hemorrhage. *Semin Neurol.* 2010;30:565–572.

Flegel WA. How I manage donors and patients with a weak D phenotype. *Curr Opin Hematol.* 2006;13:476–483.

Forgie MA, Wells PS, Laupacis A, Fergusson D. Preoperative autologous donation decreased allogeneic transfusion but increases exposure to all red blood cell transfusion: results of a meta-analysis. *Arch Intern Med.* 1998; 158:610–616.

Fresh-Frozen Plasma, Cryoprecipitate, and Platelets Administration Practice Guidelines Development Task Force of the College. Practice parameter for the use of fresh-frozen plasma, cryoprecipitate, and platelets. *JAMA.* 1994;271:777–781.

Fung K, Eason E, Crane J, et al. Prevention of Rh alloimmunization. *J Obstet Gynaecol Can.* 2003;25:765–773.

Garbe E, Andersohn F, Bronder E, et al. Drug induced immune haemolytic anaemia in the Berlin case-control surveillance study. *Br J Haematol.* 2011;154:644–653.

Garratty G. Do we need to be more concerned about weak D antigens? *Transfusion.* 2005;45:1547–1551.

Garratty G. Drug-induced immune hemolytic anemia. *Hematol Am Soc Hematol Educ Program.* 2009;1:73–79.

Garratty G, Petz LD. Approaches to selecting blood for transfusion to patients with autoimmune hemolytic anemia. *Transfusion.* 2002;42:1390–1392.

Geiger TL, Howard SC. Acetaminophen and diphenhydramine premedication for allergic and febrile nonhemolytic transfusion reactions: good prophylaxis or bad practice? *Transfus Med Rev.* 2007;21:1–12.

George JN. Clinical practice. Thrombotic thrombocytopenic purpura. *N Engl J Med.* 2006;354:1927–1935.

Gohel MS, Bulbulia RA, Slim FJ, et al. How to approach major surgery where patients refuse blood transfusion (including Jehovah's Witnesses). *Ann R Coll Surg Engl.* 2005;87:3–14.

Hérbert PC, Wells G, Blajchman MA, et al. A multicenter, randomized, controlled clinical trial of transfusion requirements in critical care. Transfusion Requirements in Critical Care Investigators, Canadian Critical Care Trials Group. *N Engl J Med.* 1999;340:409–417.

Hébert PC, Wells G, Tweeddale M, et al. Does transfusion practice affect mortality in critically ill patients? Transfusion Requirements in Critical Care (TRICC) Investigators and the Canadian Critical Care Trials Group. *Am J Respir Crit Care Med.* 1997;155:1618–1623.

Hoffmeister KM. The role of lectins and glycans in platelet clearance. *J Thromb Haemost.* 2011;9(suppl 1):35–43.

Hoffmeister KM, Flebinger TW, Falet H, et al. The clearance mechanism of chilled blood platelets. *Cell.* 2003;112:87–97.

Howard SC, Gajjar A, Ribeiro RC, et al. Safety of lumbar puncture for children with acute lymphoblastic leukemia and thrombocytopenia. *JAMA.* 2000;284:2222–2224.

Josephson CD, Mullis N, Van Demark C, Hillyer CD. Significant numbers of apheresis-derived group O platelet units have "high-titer" anti-A/A,B: implications for transfusion policy. *Transfusion.* 2004;44:805–808.

Joy SD, Rossi KQ, Krugh D, et al. Management of pregnancies complicated by anti-E alloimmunization. *Obstet Gynecol.* 2005;105:24–28.

Judd WJ. Practice guidelines for prenatal and perinatal immunohematology, revised. *Transfusion.* 2001;41:1445–1452.

Keller AJ, Chirnside A, Urbaniak SJ. Coagulation abnormalities produced by plasma exchange on the cell separator with special reference to fibrinogen and platelet levels. *Br J Haematol.* 1979;42:593–603.

Klein HG, Anstee DJ. Haemolytic disease of the fetus and newborn. In: Klein HG, Anstee DJ, eds. *Mollison's Blood Transfusion in Clinical Medicine.* 11th ed. Hoboken, NJ: Wiley-Blackwell; 2005:496–545.

Kleinman S, Caulfield T, Chan P, et al. Toward an understanding of transfusion-related acute lung injury: statement on the consensus panel. *Transfusion.* 2004;44:1774–1789.

Koelewijn JM, Vrijkotte TG, van der Schoot CE, et al. Effect of screening for red cell antibodies, other than anti-D, to detect the molytic disease of the fetus and newborn: a population study in the Netherlands. *Transfusion.* 2008;48:941–952.

Kruskall MS. The perils of platelet transfusions. *N Engl J Med.* 1997;337:1914–1915.

Kuriyan M, Fox E. Pretransfusion testing without serologic crossmatch: approaches to ensure patient safety. *Vox Sang.* 2000;78:113–118.

LaSalle-Williams M, Nuss R, Le T, et al. Extended red blood cell antigen matching for transfusions in sickle cell disease: a review of a 14-year experience from a single center. *Transfusion.* 2011;51:1732–1739.

Li G, Rachmale S, Kojicic M, et al. Incidence of transfusion risk factors for transfusion-associated circulatory overload among medical intensive care unit patients. *Transfusion.* 2011;51:338–343.

Marques MB, Huang ST. Patients with thrombotic thrombocytopenic purpura commonly develop metabolic alkalosis during therapeutic plasma exchange. *J Clin Apher.* 2001;16:120–124.

McClain CM, Patel C, Szklarski P, Booth GS. Identification of blood draw error during trauma resuscitation. *Transfusion.* 2012;52(9):1855–1856.

Mokrzycki MH, Kaplan AA. Therapeutic plasma exchange: complications and management. *Am J Kidney Dis.* 1994;23:817–827.

Morrison FS, Mollison PL. Post-transfusion purpura. *N Engl J Med.* 1966;275:243–248.

Oh H, Loberiza FR Jr, Zhang MJ, et al. Comparison of graft-versus-host-disease and survival after HLA-identical sibling bone marrow transplantation in ethnic populations. *Blood.* 2005;105:1408–1416.

O'Leary MF, Szklarski P, Klein TM, Young PP. Hemolysis of red blood cells after cell washing with different automated technologies: clinical implications in a neonatal cardiac surgery population. *Transfusion.* 2011;51: 955–960.

Osby M, Shulman IA. Phenotype matching of donor red blood cell units for nonalloimmunized sickle cell disease patients: a survey of 1182 North American laboratories. *Arch Pathol Lab Med.* 2005;129:190–193.

O'Shaughnessy DF, Atterbury C, Bolton Maggs P, et al. British Committee for Standards in Haematology, Blood Transfusion Task Force. Guidelines for the use of fresh frozen plasma, cryoprecipitate and cryosupernatant. *Br Soc Haematol.* 2004;126:11–28.

Passannante A, Macik BG. The heparin flush syndrome: a cause of iatrogenic hemorrhage. *Am J Med Sci.* 1988;296:71–73.

Rama BN, Haake RD, Bander SJ, et al. Heparin flush associated thrombocytopenia–induced hemorrhage: a case report. *Nebr Med J.* 1991;76:392–394.

Rogers DM, Crookston KP. The approach to the patient who refuses blood transfusion. *Transfusion.* 2006;46:1471–1477.

Sandler SG. How I manage patients suspected of having had an IgA anaphylactic transfusion reaction. *Transfusion.* 2006;46:10–13.

Sandler SG, Mallory D, Malamut D, Eckrich R. IgA anaphylactic transfusion reactions. *Transfus Med Rev.* 1995; 9:1–8.

Sandler SG, Zantek ND. Review: IgA anaphylactic transfusion reactions. Part II. Clinical diagnosis and bedside management. *Immunohematology.* 2004;20:234–238.

Schramm B, Leslie K, Myles PS, Hogan CJ. Coagulation studies in pre-operative neurosurgical patients. *Anesth Intensive Care.* 2001;29:388–392.

Shah J, Fitz-Henry J. Peri-operative care series. *Ann R Coll Surg Engl.* 2011;93:265–267.

Shtalrid M, Shvidel L, Vorst E, et al. Post-transfusion purpura: a challenging diagnosis. *Isr Med Assoc J.* 2006;8:672–674.

Slichter SJ, Davis K, Enright H, et al. Factors affecting post-transfusion platelet increments, platelet refractoriness, and platelet transfusion intervals in thrombocytopenic patients. *Blood.* 2005;105:4106–4114.

Smith HM, Farrow SJ, Ackerman JD, et al. Cardiac arrests associated with hyperkalemia during red blood cell transfusion: a case series. *Anesth Analg.* 2008;106:1062–1069.

Sokol RJ, Booker DJ, Stamps R. The pathology of autoimmune hemolytic anemia. *J Clin Pathol.* 1992;45:1047–1052.

Sokol RJ, Hewitt S, Stamps BK. Autoimmune hemolysis: an 18-year study of 865 cases referred to a regional transfusion center. *Br Med J (Clin Res Ed).* 1981;282:2023–2027.

Squires JE. Risks of transfusion. *South Med J.* 2011;104(11): 762–769.

Stehling LC, Doherty DC, Faust RJ, et al. Practice guidelines for blood component therapy: a report by the American Society of Anesthesiologists Task Force on Blood Component Therapy. *Anesthesiology.* 1996;84:732–747.

Stephens LC, Haire WD, Tatantolo S, et al. Normal saline versus heparin flush for maintaining central venous catheter patency during apheresis collection of peripheral blood stem cells (PBSC). *Transfus Sci.* 1997;18:187–193.

Tormey CA, Stack G. The persistence and evanescence of blood group alloantibodies in men. *Transfusion.* 2009;49:505–512.

Toy P, Gajic O, Bacchetti P, et al. Transfusion-related acute lung injury: incidence and risk factors. *Blood.* 2012;119(7):1757–1767.

Vamvakas EC, Pineda AA, Reisner R, et al. The differentiation of delayed hemolytic and delayed serologic transfusion reactions: incidence and predictors of hemolysis. *Transfusion.* 1995;35:26–32.

Vaughn JI, Manning M, Warwick RM, et al. Inhibition of erythroid progenitor cells by anti-Kell antibodies in fetal alloimmune anemia. *N Engl J Med.* 1998;338:798–803.

Vichinsky EP, Luban NL, Wright E, et al. Prospective RBC phenotype matching in a stroke-prevention trial in sickle cell anemia: a multicenter transfusion trial. *Transfusion.* 2001;41:1086–1092.

Weinstein R. Hypocalcemic toxicity and atypical reactions in therapeutic plasma exchange. *J Clin Apher.* 2001;16:210–211.

Whitlock RP, Sun JC, Fremes SE, et al. Antithrombotic and thrombolytic therapy for valvular disease: antithrombotic therapy and prevention of thrombosis, 9th ed: American College of Chest Physicians evidence-based clinical practice guidelines. *Chest.* 2012;141(2 suppl): e576S–e600S.

Wieling W, France CR, van Dijk N, et al. Physiologic strategies to prevent fainting responses during or after whole blood donation. *Transfusion.* 2011;51:2727–2738.

Wynn RF, Stevens RF, Bolton-Maggs PH, et al. Paroxysmal cold hemoglobinuria of childhood: a review of the management and unusual presenting features of six cases. *Clin Lab Hematol.* 1998;20:373–375.

Yeh JH, Chiu HC. Coagulation abnormalities in serial double-filtration plasmapheresis. *J Clin Apher.* 2001;16:139–142.

Zeidler K, Arn K, Senn O, et al. Optimal preprocedural platelet transfusion threshold for central venous catheter insertions in patients with thrombocytopenia. *Transfusion.* 2011;51:2269–2276.

CHAPTER 2
Coagulation Disorders

MICHAEL LAPOSATA

MONITORING OF ANTICOAGULANT THERAPY IN PATIENTS BEING TREATED WITH WARFARIN

Errors in anticoagulation therapy have become a major source of concern to hospital accrediting agencies. The simple error of not knowing about an elevated international normalized ratio (INR) value and therefore not taking an appropriate action is very common. Another common adverse outcome in warfarin-treated patients occurs from inappropriate decisions about dosing of warfarin, because many clinicians do not know the appropriate response to a supratherapeutic or subtherapeutic INR value. Such errors can result in catastrophic bleeding or thrombosis that is preventable. The laboratory can also contribute to error if it fails to use the correct formula for generation of the INR value.

TEST ORDERING MISTAKES

- *Ordering the INR too soon after the initiation of warfarin therapy*. The effect of warfarin occurs several days after the therapy is initiated. Checking the INR in the first three days of the administration of warfarin could lead to an inappropriate adjustment of the warfarin dose.

Not checking the INR value at least once per month. The maximum time interval for checking the INR value in a warfarin-treated patient is once per month, although there have been recent suggestions to lengthen this period in highly stable patients. Data now show the benefit of patients performing home testing for the INR. A meta-analysis revealed that patients who measure their own INR with a point of care device at home perform the INR two to four times more frequently than they would if they were managed by their physicians. Importantly, home-monitored patients with more frequent testing experience less bleeding and less thrombosis.

Determining the effect of warfarin reversal with vitamin K too soon. Many variables influence the time to reduction in INR with vitamin K therapy. For patients treated with oral vitamin K at a dose of 1 to 5 mg orally, the expectation is that a reduction in INR will occur within 24 hours; for intravenously delivered vitamin K, a reduction in the INR should be observed even sooner, typically within 12 hours.

MISTAKES IN RESULT INTERPRETATION

Failing to review and act upon an INR value in a timely fashion. One of the most common mistakes occurs when the physician is unaware of an elevated INR value. This often happens when one physician is cross covering the patients of another physician and is unaware of the clinical status of the warfarin-treated patient for whom he or she has assumed temporary responsibility.

Misunderstanding the clinical significance of an elevated INR value. Generally speaking, if there is a concern of serious bleeding in a warfarin-treated patient with a markedly elevated INR, usually above 10, fresh frozen plasma along with vitamin K needs to be administered to rapidly reverse the warfarin effect. Other approaches are available for replacement of factors II, VII, IX, and X. These involve the use of prothrombin complex concentrates containing these four factors and the use of recombinant factor VIIa. Bleeding that does not appear to be life threatening can be treated with oral vitamin K. Mildly elevated INR values can be treated by the temporary discontinuation of warfarin. In addition, an INR value significantly below the therapeutic range needs to be treated with an increase in the warfarin dose. In all cases, a thorough investigation for the cause of any supratherapeutic or subtherapeutic INR must be performed.

Interpreting the INR value without qualification in the presence of interfering factors. One such example is for a patient receiving both argatroban and warfarin, with the goal of discontinuing the argatroban and continuing the warfarin long term. A therapeutic dose of argatroban will significantly elevate the INR in all patients. The INR value in the presence of argatroban should not be used to determine whether the patient is effectively anticoagulated with warfarin. Options include removing the argatroban for 2 to 3 hours and testing at that time with the INR or using a chromogenic factor X assay to monitor warfarin as this test does not suffer interference by argatroban.

OTHER MISTAKES

Failure of the laboratory to appropriately calculate the INR from the prothrombin time (PT) values generated from the patient samples. One of the major problems uncovered in clinical laboratories over the past decade is the incorrect calculation of the INR value. One cause for this incorrect calculation in some laboratories is that the value for the international sensitivity index (ISI) has been incorrectly assigned for the reagents in use to perform the PT assay, from which the INR is calculated.

CONTROVERSIES

- *Using the INR as a replacement value for the PT in patients not receiving warfarin.* The INR value is derived using data from patients who are being treated with warfarin. These patients have specific factor deficiencies (low levels of factors II, VII, IX, and X) that are a result of warfarin therapy. The clinical laboratory cannot easily know whether a sample for a PT test is from a warfarin-treated patient or a patient with liver disease, for example. Because there is a need to convert the PT value to an INR in the warfarin-treated patient, laboratory information systems typically convert all PT values into INR values. The clinicians then see values for both the PT and the INR for all patients for whom a PT test has been requested. The clinical use of the INR instead of the PT for nonwarfarinized patients was originally discouraged. However, the INR appears to be an effective surrogate test for the PT, and now many clinicians follow the INR rather than the PT for patients with, for example, liver disease and disseminated intravascular coagulation (DIC).
- *There is substantial controversy about the merits of pharmacogenomic testing to assess for warfarin sensitivity.* The FDA supports such testing, but the logistical challenge is very high to determine the status of CYP2C9 (eg, 3*/3* genotype patients should be treated with a lower warfarin dose) and vitamin K epoxide reductase (VKORC1, the AA genotype patients benefit from a lower warfarin dose) within the first few days of warfarin therapy and permit early dose adjustment. There is now

significant data to show that pharmacogenomic testing for warfarin sensitivity shortens the time to stable dosing and increases the time that patients receiving warfarin are within the therapeutic range.

STANDARDS OF CARE

- Patients receiving warfarin must be monitored using the INR. Warfarin dose adjustment should not occur until the patient has received two to three doses of warfarin and monitoring should occur at least once per month.
- Subtherapeutic and supratherapeutic INR values must be acted upon in a timely fashion to minimize the risk of bleeding or thrombosis. Values that are substantially outside the therapeutic range require immediate attention to prevent a potentially lethal outcome.
- When the INR does not reflect the effect of warfarin alone, but is confounded by other variables, warfarin dose adjustment must take into account such confounders.
- The laboratory must correctly calculate the INR from the PT value of the patient.

MONITORING OF ANTICOAGULANT THERAPY IN PATIENTS BEING TREATED WITH UNFRACTIONATED HEPARIN

Patients receiving unfractionated heparin are most commonly monitored using the partial thromboplastin time (PTT) assay. However, many clinical laboratories monitoring heparin-treated patients are now using an assay for anti-factor Xa. There is substantial variability in patient response to unfractionated heparin therapy. In addition, the laboratory reagent used in the performance of the PTT shows lot-to-lot variability, and this can introduce substantial analytical variability in the PTT. Thus, the biological and the analytical variability associated with heparin treatment make it difficult to continuously maintain a patient within the therapeutic PTT range. As with all anticoagulants, errors surrounding anticoagulation therapy have become highly visible because they can result in catastrophic bleeding or thrombosis, and they are often preventable. Another major complication associated with heparin therapy is the development of heparin-induced thrombocytopenia (HIT) with thrombosis. Monitoring the platelet count in a hospitalized patient on intravenous unfractionated heparin therapy is essential to reduce the incidence of this potentially lethal thrombotic condition by discontinuing heparin therapy and introducing an anticoagulant unrelated to heparin.

TEST ORDERING MISTAKES

■ *Not ordering a platelet count at least every third day while a patient is in the hospital receiving unfractionated heparin, as an assessment for HIT.*

■ *Requesting an anti-factor Xa assay to monitor the effect of unfractionated heparin, but not indicating to the laboratory that the test is assessing the effect of unfractionated heparin.* Low molecular weight heparin is also monitored by an anti-factor Xa assay. The laboratory uses unfractionated heparin to calibrate the assay when the anticoagulant effect of unfractionated heparin is being assessed; and it uses low molecular weight heparin when the anticoagulant effect of low molecular weight heparin is being assessed. The laboratory must know, therefore, whether the test request is for the assessment of anticoagulation with unfractionated heparin or low molecular weight heparin.

MISTAKES IN RESULT INTERPRETATION

▨ *Failing to review and act upon a supratherapeutic or subtherapeutic PTT value in a patient being treated with unfractionated heparin value in a timely fashion.* The consequences for a patient requiring anticoagulation with unfractionated heparin whose PTT is not in the therapeutic range are bleeding (for PTT values above the therapeutic range) and thrombosis (for PTT values below the therapeutic range). The bleeding or thrombotic events can range from mild to lethal, and for that reason, maintenance of the heparin-treated patient within the therapeutic PTT range greatly improves patient outcome.

▨ *Failing to pursue a diagnosis of HIT upon observing a decline in the platelet count to 50% or less of the baseline platelet count, in a patient exposed to unfractionated heparin or low molecular weight heparin by any route and at any dose, particularly in the absence of an alternative explanation for the decrease in platelets.*

▨ *Concluding that the PTT is within the therapeutic range in a patient receiving heparin, who also has a lupus anticoagulant or other condition associated with a prolonged PTT, such as factor XII deficiency.* Using the lupus anticoagulant as an example, the lupus anticoagulant can prolong the PTT. However, this prolongation is not reflective of an anticoagulation effect. If a patient with a lupus anticoagulant develops thrombosis and requires treatment with heparin, and the PTT is already elevated above the upper limit of normal before heparin treatment, the patient may receive an inadequate amount of heparin if the physician uses the standard PTT therapeutic range to adjust heparin dosing. In such cases, the PTT cannot be used to assess the effectiveness of anticoagulation with heparin. The anti-factor Xa assay for unfractionated heparin must be used in these cases. Providing a thrombotic patient with an inadequate dose of unfractionated heparin can result in clinically significant thrombosis.

■ *Confusing the therapeutic range in the anti-factor Xa assay for unfractionated heparin (0.3–0.7 U/mL) with that of the therapeutic range for low molecular weight heparin (0.5–1.0 U/mL).*

■ *Expecting a therapeutic PTT or a therapeutic anti-factor Xa level after treatment with prophylactic unfractionated heparin doses, commonly 5,000 units two or three times per day.* Prophylactic doses do not produce a therapeutic levels unless there is a confounding variable also prolonging the PTT.

OTHER MISTAKES

■ *Samples from heparinized patients in whole blood will have a declining PTT value as they remain in whole blood for several hours before the analysis.* Activation of even a small percentage of the platelets in whole blood results in the release of a substance from the activated platelets that neutralize heparin. The clinical impact of this preanalytical error is that the patient may have a therapeutic PTT in vivo that is inappropriately observed to be subtherapeutic, or a supratherapeutic PTT that is incorrectly perceived as therapeutic. The clinical impact of either of the situations is incorrect heparin dosing of the patient. A standard recommendation is that a whole-blood specimen is processed to separate blood cells from plasma within 4 hours of sample collection.

CONTROVERSIES

■ *There is substantial controversy for patients receiving unfractionated heparin on whether the use of the anti-factor Xa assay for monitoring unfractionated heparin is more reflective of bleeding and thrombotic risk than the PTT.* The assay for anti-factor Xa in the clinical laboratory is much more expensive than the PTT, and it is also more complex and therefore requires more sophisticated instrumentation than the PTT.

These limitations notwithstanding, many clinical laboratories have instituted heparin monitoring with anti-factor Xa assays.

STANDARDS OF CARE

▪ Patients receiving unfractionated heparin must be monitored for bleeding and thrombotic complications using either a therapeutic PTT range or a therapeutic anti-factor Xa range for unfractionated heparin. Supratherapeutic and subtherapeutic PTT or anti-factor Xa values must be acted upon in a timely fashion to minimize the risk of bleeding or thrombosis.

▪ Patients receiving unfractionated heparin, especially those in the hospital, should be monitored for the development of HIT with platelet counts at least every third day.

▪ Patients who have a prolonged PTT before the initiation of heparin therapy cannot be monitored with the PTT assay to determine heparin dosing. An anti-factor Xa assay must be used in these cases, with careful attention to use the therapeutic range associated with unfractionated heparin and not low molecular weight heparin.

▪ Specimens to be evaluated with a PTT assay to assess the effect of heparin anticoagulation must be processed to separate plasma from blood cells within 4 hours of collection to avoid preanalytical neutralization of heparin in the specimen.

MONITORING OF ANTICOAGULANT THERAPY IN PATIENTS BEING TREATED WITH LOW MOLECULAR WEIGHT HEPARIN

Unlike unfractionated heparin, the biological and analytical variability associated with low molecular weight heparin treatment is highly reproducible. For this reason, it is unnecessary to monitor the anticoagulation effect of low molecular weight heparin in most patients. For those patients who do need monitoring (see section Result Interpretation Mistakes for indications), the appropriate test is the anti-factor Xa assay. As with all anticoagulants, errors surrounding anticoagulation therapy have become highly visible, because such errors can result in catastrophic bleeding or thrombosis, and they are often preventable. Although it is less common in patients receiving low molecular weight heparin than unfractionated heparin, a serious complication associated with low molecular weight heparin therapy is the development of HIT with thrombosis. The platelet count in patients receiving low molecular weight heparin, for several compelling reasons described in this chapter, is monitored less often than it is for hospitalized patients receiving unfractionated heparin.

TEST ORDERING MISTAKES

- *Ordering a PTT assay to monitor anticoagulation with low molecular weight heparin instead of the anti-factor Xa assay.* Low molecular weight heparin treatment, even at therapeutic doses, results in only a mild prolongation of the PTT in most cases.
- *Requesting an anti-factor Xa assay to monitor the effect of low molecular weight heparin, but not indicating to the laboratory that the test is assessing the effect of low molecular weight heparin.* Unfractionated heparin is also monitored by an anti-factor Xa assay. The laboratory uses low molecular weight heparin to calibrate the assay when the anticoagulant effect of low molecular weight heparin is being assessed, and it uses unfractionated heparin when the anticoagulant effect of unfractionated heparin is being assessed. The laboratory must know, therefore, whether the test request is assessing anticoagulation with low molecular weight heparin or unfractionated heparin.

MISTAKES IN RESULT INTERPRETATION

▨ *Failing to review and act upon a supratherapeutic or sub-therapeutic anti-factor Xa value in a patient being treated with low molecular weight heparin in a timely fashion.* This applies only to patients who have a requirement for being monitored while receiving low molecular weight heparin. The majority of patients receiving low molecular weight heparin do not require monitoring with any assay to assess the extent of anticoagulation. Indications for monitoring include renal impairment; elevated body mass index; low body mass index; pregnancy; infancy, especially in the neonatal period; and long-term anticoagulation with low molecular weight heparin. The consequences for patients requiring anticoagulation with low molecular weight heparin whose anti-factor Xa is not in the therapeutic range are bleeding (for anti-factor Xa values above the therapeutic range) and thrombosis (for anti-factor Xa values below the therapeutic range). As with all anticoagulants, the bleeding or thrombotic events can range from mild to lethal, and for this reason maintenance of the patient treated with low molecular weight heparin within the therapeutic anti-factor Xa range is absolutely essential.

▨ *Failing to pursue a diagnosis of HIT upon a decline in the platelet count to 50% or less of the baseline platelet count in a patient exposed to low molecular weight heparin by any route at any dose, in the absence of an alternative explanation for the decrease in platelets.* Although unfractionated heparin is more frequently associated with HIT, exposure to low molecular weight heparin alone can produce HIT.

▨ *Confusing the therapeutic range in the anti-factor Xa assay for low molecular weight heparin (0.5–1.0 U/mL) with that of unfractionated heparin (0.3–0.7 U/mL).*

▨ *Expecting a therapeutic anti-factor Xa level after treatment with prophylactic low molecular weight heparin doses.* Treatment with prophylactic doses of low molecular weight heparin produces anti-factor Xa levels that are well below the therapeutic range.

OTHER MISTAKES

Not collecting a blood sample for anti-factor Xa monitoring of the patient treated with low molecular weight heparin at 4 hours after subcutaneous administration of the low molecular weight heparin. The therapeutic effect of low molecular weight heparin is assessed at 4 hours postinjection. Values before and after 4 hours (within a window of about 15–30 minutes) will be different from those obtained at 4 hours, and the misleading laboratory result could lead to inappropriate adjustment of the low molecular weight heparin dose.

Whole-blood samples from patients treated with low molecular weight heparin will show a declining anti-factor Xa value as the time between sample collection and analysis is increased. For this reason, whole-blood samples must be centrifuged to separate the blood cells from the plasma. Activation of even a small percentage of the platelets in whole blood results in the release of platelet factor 4 from the activated platelets, which neutralizes heparin and low molecular weight heparin. The clinical impact of this preanalytical error is that the patient may have a therapeutic anti-factor Xa in vivo that is inappropriately deemed subtherapeutic, or have a true supratherapeutic anti-factor Xa that is incorrectly perceived as therapeutic. The clinical impact of either of the situations is incorrect dosing of the patient with low molecular weight heparin. As with unfractionated heparin, a standard recommendation is that a whole-blood specimen is processed to separate blood cells from plasma within 4 hours of sample collection.

CONTROVERSIES

Not ordering a platelet count at least every third day for the patient receiving low molecular weight heparin, at least while a patient is in the hospital, and not beginning platelet count checks on the fourth day following initial heparin exposure, as an assessment for HIT. Although monitoring the platelet count for patients receiving unfractionated heparin in the hospital to assess for HIT is well accepted, monitoring the platelet count for patients receiving low molecular weight heparin is controversial. This is because low molecular weight heparin is often given for treatment of outpatients, and it is more difficult to test outpatients than inpatients, especially on a regular basis, for the platelet count. In addition, the risk for development of HIT after exposure to low molecular weight heparin is less than it is for unfractionated heparin. Finally, there is appropriate widespread use of prophylactic anticoagulation of hospitalized patients with low molecular weight heparin to prevent thrombosis. Monitoring of platelet counts in this population would require platelet counts of a large number of hospitalized patients. Generally speaking, many experts would consider it advisable to monitor the platelet count at some point during hospitalization for a patient receiving therapeutic doses of low molecular weight heparin.

STANDARDS OF CARE

- Patients receiving low molecular weight heparin who must be monitored for bleeding and thrombotic complications are evaluated using an anti-factor Xa assay with a therapeutic range for low molecular weight heparin of 0.5 to 1.0 U/mL.
- Subtherapeutic and supratherapeutic anti-factor Xa values must be acted upon in a timely fashion to minimize the risk of bleeding or thrombosis. Values that are substantially outside the therapeutic range require immediate attention to prevent a potentially lethal outcome.

▦ Although it is controversial, it is a safe practice for patients receiving low molecular weight heparin, especially those in the hospital and who are receiving treatment doses of low molecular weight heparin, to be screened for the development of HIT with platelet counts at some point.

▦ For monitoring the effect of low molecular weight heparin with an anti-factor Xa assay, samples must be collected 4 hours after the subcutaneous injection of low molecular weight heparin. Dosing of low molecular weight heparin is based on the value collected at this time, and dose adjustment based on results of samples collected more than 30 minutes before or after 4 hours may be incorrect.

▦ Whole-blood specimens to be evaluated with an anti-factor Xa assay to assess the effect of low molecular weight heparin anticoagulation must be processed to separate plasma from blood cells within 4 hours of collection to avoid the preanalytical neutralization of low molecular weight heparin in the specimen.

MONITORING OF ANTICOAGULANT THERAPY IN PATIENTS BEING TREATED WITH FONDAPARINUX

Fondaparinux is a pentasaccharide that is chemically synthesized, unlike unfractionated heparin and its derivative low molecular weight heparin, which are derived from pig intestine. Its pharmacokinetics is so reproducible in nearly all patients with adequate renal function that it is rarely necessary to monitor its anticoagulation effect. The reproducibility of the pharmacologic effect is comparable to or better than that found for low molecular weight heparin. For those patients who do require monitoring, the appropriate test is the anti-factor Xa assay. Patients who have moderate to severe renal impairment must not receive this anticoagulant, as it is cleared exclusively by the kidney. Monitoring may be highly informative in a patient with renal disease who inappropriately received fondaparinux and begins to bleed.

Importantly, fondaparinux has no well-established reversibility agent. Protamine sulfate can be used to neutralize unfractionated heparin and much of the activity of low molecular weight heparin, but it does not neutralize fondaparinux. In addition, the half-life for fondaparinux is on the order of 20 hours, unlike low molecular weight heparin with a half-life of about 5 hours and unfractionated heparin with a half-life of approximately 1 hour. It is extremely rare to identify a fondaparinux-treated patient who has a clinically significant complication of HIT. Monitoring the platelet count in patients receiving fondaparinux, therefore, is not indicated.

TEST ORDERING MISTAKES

Failing to measure the creatinine or other assessment of renal function before administering fondaparinux.

Requesting an anti-factor Xa assay to monitor the effect of fondaparinux, but not indicating to the laboratory that the test is assessing the effect of fondaparinux. Unfractionated heparin and low molecular weight heparin can also be monitored by an anti-factor Xa assay. The laboratory uses fondaparinux to calibrate the assay when the anticoagulant effect of fondaparinux is being assessed; it uses low molecular weight heparin to calibrate the assay when the anticoagulant effect of low molecular weight heparin is being assessed; and it uses unfractionated heparin when the anticoagulant effect of unfractionated heparin is being measured. The laboratory must be made aware, therefore, that the requested test is to monitor the effect of fondaparinux.

MISTAKES IN RESULT INTERPRETATION

Failing to review and act upon a supratherapeutic or subtherapeutic anti-factor Xa value in a patient being treated with fondaparinux in a timely fashion. The potential consequences for patients requiring anticoagulation with fondaparinux whose anti-factor Xa is not in the therapeutic range are bleeding (for anti-factor Xa values above the therapeutic range) and thrombosis (for anti-factor Xa values below the therapeutic range).

Confusing the therapeutic range in the anti-factor Xa assay for fondaparinux (0.5–1.5 U/mL for a 7.5 mg daily dose) with that of the range for low molecular weight heparin (0.5–1.0 U/mL) and unfractionated heparin (0.3–0.7 U/mL).

Expecting a therapeutic anti-factor Xa level after treatment with a prophylactic fondaparinux dose. Treatment with a prophylactic dose of fondaparinux produces an anti-factor Xa level that is well below the therapeutic range.

OTHER MISTAKES

Not collecting a sample for anti-factor Xa monitoring of the patient treated with fondaparinux at the correct time after subcutaneous administration of the drug. The therapeutic effect of fondaparinux should be assessed after at least 3 hours post injection. Values before 3 hours may be different from those obtained after 3 hours. The half-life for fondaparinux is relatively long, so the timing of the blood sampling need not be as precise as for monitoring low molecular weight heparin. A misleading laboratory result could lead to inappropriate adjustment of the fondaparinux dose. It should be noted, however, that dosing of fondaparinux is not as precise as dosing of low molecular weight heparin. Patients less than 50 kg are recommended to receive 5 mg of fondaparinux daily; patients weighing between 50 and 100 kg are recommended to receive 7.5 mg of fondaparinux daily; and patients weighing more than 100 kg should receive 10 mg daily. Dosing with low molecular weight heparin is on a per kilogram basis, as is dosing with unfractionated heparin. Therefore, dose adjustments are far more commonly required with unfractionated heparin and low molecular weight heparin than for fondaparinux.

CONTROVERSIES

It is not absolutely clear whether treatment with fondaparinux carries any risk for development of clinically significant HIT. There have been case reports of an occasional patient who may have developed HIT following exposure to fondaparinux. Importantly, if these patients had any previous exposure to heparin or low molecular weight heparin in any form at any time, which was not known to the authors of these reports, fondaparinux may not have been the cause of the observed HIT.

STANDARDS OF CARE

- Patients receiving fondaparinux who must be monitored for bleeding and thrombotic complications are evaluated using an anti-factor Xa assay with a therapeutic range for fondaparinux of 0.5 to 1.5 U/mL for patients receiving 7.5 mg of fondaparinux daily.
- Subtherapeutic and supratherapeutic anti-factor Xa values must be recognized in a timely fashion, though it may be difficult to minimize the risk of bleeding if the value is supratherapeutic because there is no reversal agent for fondaparinux.
- Samples collected for monitoring the effect of fondaparinux with an anti-factor Xa assay must not be collected before 3 hours from the time of the subcutaneous injection of the drug.

MONITORING OF ANTICOAGULANT THERAPY IN PATIENTS BEING TREATED WITH ARGATROBAN

Direct thrombin inhibitors, which include argatroban, are commonly used anticoagulants in patients with HIT and in individuals tested for whatever reason and found to have antibodies to the heparin–platelet factor 4 complex in the absence of thrombocytopenia or thrombosis. Argatroban is monitored with the standard PTT assay. Monitoring is especially important because argatroban has no effective antidote to reverse over-anticoagulation. Monitoring is also made more difficult because argatroban also has an effect on the PT and, as a result, on the INR derived from it. In a typical patient with HIT transitioning from argatroban to warfarin, in an overlap phase during which time warfarin is present along with argatroban, there are special considerations necessary to obtain an INR that accurately reflects warfarin-induced anticoagulation. In addition, frequent monitoring of the PTT is highly recommended, especially if argatroban is used in the presence of liver dysfunction.

TEST ORDERING MISTAKES

- *Not monitoring the PTT frequently enough after the initiation of therapy with argatroban.* Argatroban is cleared by the liver, and, therefore, liver disease can reduce the rate at which argatroban is removed from the circulation. It is common to use argatroban in patients with liver disease, but at a reduced dose. In patients with liver disease, monitoring of the PTT more than once per day to determine if the standard argatroban dose has been correctly reduced is essential to avoid under- or over-anticoagulation of the patient.
- *Argatroban produces significant interference with the INR. Therefore, in patients being treated with*

argatroban and warfarin at the same time, with the intention to discontinue argatroban when a therapeutic effect of warfarin is achieved, the INR cannot be used to determine the warfarin effect. In such cases, the argatroban can be discontinued for 2 to 3 hours (the half-life is approximately 20 minutes), and the INR tested at that time. Because the patient might not be therapeutically anticoagulated with warfarin, the removal of argatroban can result in thrombosis during this interval. Another option is to use a chromogenic assay for factor X to determine if warfarin has decreased the level of factor X to an expected concentration. Warfarin typically decreases factor X, along with factors II, VII, and IX. The chromogenic assay for factor X is not affected by argatroban. This permits testing for a warfarin effect while the patient is still receiving argatroban, and thereby anticoagulated with argatroban even if the warfarin effect is subtherapeutic at that time. A chromogenic factor X level of less than 45% has been recommended as adequate to permit discontinuation of argatroban and treatment with warfarin alone.

MISTAKES IN RESULT INTERPRETATION

▨ *Underdosing argatroban in patients with both HIT and the lupus anticoagulant.* In the rare patient with both HIT and a lupus anticoagulant, the PTT is prolonged before anticoagulation from the lupus anticoagulant. If the standard target range for argatroban of 1.5 to 2.5 times the mean of the normal PTT range is used to dose the argatroban, an inadequate dose of the anticoagulant is likely to be provided. If the PT is not prolonged from the lupus anticoagulant, an increase in the PT to an arbitrarily accepted therapeutic range is one option to monitor argatroban in these circumstances.

STANDARDS OF CARE

- Patients receiving argatroban should be monitored more than once per day, especially as the anticoagulant dose is adjusted and when argatroban is used in patients with liver disease.
- Patients being treated with argatroban and warfarin should ideally be monitored to assess warfarin-induced anticoagulation with a chromogenic factor X assay. Another option is to discontinue the argatroban for 2 to 3 hours and then perform the INR to assess the warfarin effect.
- Patients with both HIT and a lupus anticoagulant that prolongs the PTT, being treated with argatroban, cannot being monitored with the standard target PTT range for the direct thrombin inhibitor's anticoagulation.

EVALUATION FOR HEPARIN-INDUCED THROMBOCYTOPENIA

HIT is a highly prothrombotic condition, which can lead to arterial or venous thrombosis. A diagnosis of HIT indicates that antibodies are present to the heparin–platelet factor 4 complex; and thrombocytopenia exists to less than 50% of the patient's baseline platelet count, or there is a documented thrombosis. The thrombocytopenia in this condition is relatively modest, with values in the range of 40,000 to 80,000 per microliter. Importantly, the platelet count may not be decreased below the reference range. A patient who suffers a decline in platelet count from 600,000 to 300,000 per microliter has an equivalent risk for thrombosis as someone whose platelet count decreases from 150,000 to 75,000 per microliter. If the patient's platelet count decreases less than four days after exposure to heparin, it is unlikely that the patient has HIT. The criteria known as the 4 T's to aid in the diagnosis of HIT refer to an appropriate level of Thrombocytopenia, appropriate Timing of the decline in the platelet count, the presence of Thrombosis, and the presence of oTher causes for thrombocytopenia.

HIT-associated thromboses include deep vein thrombosis, pulmonary embolism, stroke, peripheral artery thrombosis, and massive thrombosis with death. These poor clinical outcomes have in recent years resulted in a high vigilance state among physicians for this condition. There has been increased legal action against physicians who fail to recognize, demonstrate, and appropriately treat patients with HIT. The major challenge in this condition is that many patients will develop the antibody associated with HIT, which recognizes the heparin–platelet factor 4 complex, but they will not go on to develop thrombocytopenia or subsequently, thrombosis. The most commonly performed laboratory test for HIT is an enzyme-linked immunoassay, and recent improvements to this assay may better identify those patients who are at higher risk for thrombosis. Enzyme-linked immunoassays that detect immunoglobulin G (IgG) antibodies specific to the heparin–platelet factor 4 complex have a high negative predictive value. IgG antibodies activate platelets in HIT, whereas IgM antibodies do not. In addition, IgM antibodies to the heparin–platelet factor 4 complex do not precede the appearance of IgG antibodies to the same target antigen. The best evidence for a diagnosis of HIT is a functional assay with washed platelets, and it is often used to confirm a diagnosis of HIT and better identify those patients with the antibody to the heparin–platelet factor 4 complex who will go on to develop thrombosis. This complex assay involving the use of radioactive serotonin is performed in very few clinical laboratories. The lack of availability of this assay in all but a few laboratories has made it impossible to use this test to make timely decisions regarding HIT diagnosis and therapy.

Because thrombocytopenia precedes thrombosis in HIT patients in the vast majority of cases, the platelet count is the major indicator that a patient with the antibody to the heparin–platelet factor 4 complex has an elevated thrombotic risk. The concern for both the high morbidity and mortality and the legal risk for missing a diagnosis of HIT has led to overtesting for antibodies to the heparin–platelet factor 4 complex. Overtesting commonly occurs in cases in which there is only a modest decline in the platelet count. Some physicians order the test for the antibody to the heparin–platelet factor 4 complex without performing a platelet count simply because of anticipated exposure to unfractionated heparin, and the fear that a previously acquired HIT associated antibody will initiate massive thrombosis. In some circumstances, such as the postoperative state following cardiac or vascular surgery, the platelet count decreases as part of the response to surgery and cannot be used effectively as an indicator of thrombotic risk. In situations when the platelet count cannot be used as an indicator of thrombotic risk, and an antibody to the heparin–platelet factor 4 complex is present, the concern for thrombosis commonly leads to the use of anticoagulants other than unfractionated heparin or low molecular weight heparin.

TEST ORDERING MISTAKES

Failing to monitor the platelet count at least every third day in a hospitalized patient starting four days after the initial exposure to unfractionated heparin. The platelet count should be checked in patients who have had any exposure to unfractionated heparin, even if it is not provided as intravenous therapy. The platelet count can also decline, and antibodies to the heparin–platelet factor 4 complex can arise, in patients treated with low molecular weight heparin who have not been previously exposed to unfractionated heparin. However, the likelihood for the development of such antibodies is much less than that for patients exposed to unfractionated heparin.

■ *Ordering the test for antibodies to the heparin–platelet factor 4 complex when there is no meaningful decrease in platelet count (meaningful is less than 50% of baseline) and no thrombosis.* A positive test result in this assay typically forces a change to an anticoagulant other than unfractionated heparin and low molecular weight heparin, and these are more expensive and less reversible anticoagulants.

■ *Failing to order a test for antibodies to the heparin–platelet factor 4 complex in a nonthrombotic patient who has been exposed to unfractionated heparin or low molecular weight heparin who demonstrates (a) a decrease in platelet count to a level expected with HIT (approximately 50,000 per microliter as a mean value), (b) in a time frame consistent with antibody production following exposure to heparin or low molecular weight heparin (4–15 days is common in the absence of an anamnestic response), and (c) no other apparent cause for thrombocytopenia.*

MISTAKES IN RESULT INTERPRETATION

■ *Failing to completely discontinue exposure to heparin and low molecular weight heparin in a patient who has antibodies to the heparin–platelet factor 4 complex, and failing to change the anticoagulation regimen to minimize the risk for thrombosis in such patients.* Typically, this involves a change to an anticoagulant other than unfractionated heparin or low molecular weight heparin and avoidance of monotherapy with warfarin until the platelet count rises into the reference range.

■ *Treating a patient with platelets who has a positive test for antibodies to the heparin–platelet factor 4 complex.* In such patients, the antibodies can induce the generation of platelet aggregates large enough to occlude major arteries, and the transfusion of platelets increases the risk for such catastrophic thromboses.

OTHER MISTAKES

■ *The failure of the laboratory to provide the results for the test for antibodies to the heparin–platelet factor 4 complex in a timely fashion*. Delay in the processing of samples for this test forces the treating physician observing a decrease in platelet count consistent with HIT to decide whether to switch to more expensive anticoagulant therapy without a knowledge of the test results. The practical challenge for small laboratories is that the test for antibodies to the heparin–platelet factor 4 complex is often not performed on-site, but is sent to an outside laboratory. It is not uncommon in these situations to wait several days for a test result, despite the fact that there is an urgent need in such cases to make a major decision about appropriate anticoagulant use.

CONTROVERSIES

■ *Monitoring the platelet count of patients who are not in the hospital and are receiving low molecular weight heparin at home*. These patients are at some measurable risk for HIT, although it varies to some extent with their underlying clinical circumstances. For example, patients recovering from orthopedic surgery are at higher risk for development of antibodies to the heparin–platelet factor 4 complex than are patients with nonsurgical conditions. The logistical challenge of obtaining platelet counts for patients at home receiving low molecular weight heparin has resulted in acceptance of low molecular weight heparin treatment in the absence of platelet counts.

STANDARDS OF CARE

■ A platelet count should be performed at least every third day in a hospitalized patient receiving unfractionated heparin beginning four days after initial heparin exposure.

▦ A test for antibodies to the heparin–platelet factor 4 complex should be performed for a patient who has been exposed to unfractionated heparin or low molecular weight heparin and who demonstrates a decrease in platelet count that could be indicative of HIT.

▦ A test for antibodies to the heparin–platelet factor 4 complex should not be ordered when there is no meaningful decrease in platelet count (ie, less than 50% of baseline) and no thrombosis.

▦ Exposure to heparin and low molecular weight heparin must be immediately discontinued in a patient who has antibodies to the heparin–platelet factor 4 complex.

▦ The anticoagulation regimen in a patient with antibodies to the heparin–platelet factor 4 complex must be appropriate to minimize the risk for thrombosis.

▦ Platelet transfusions must be avoided in a patient who has a positive test for antibodies to the heparin–platelet factor 4 complex.

EVALUATION OF PROLONGATIONS OF THE PT AND THE PTT AND ASSESSMENT FOR DEFICIENCIES OF COAGULATION FACTORS

There are many errors associated with the orders for coagulation factors. PT and PTT prolongations may be a result of congenital deficiencies of one or more coagulation factors or from a host of acquired conditions associated with inhibitors or low levels of the coagulation factors. It is essential to diagnose the cause of a prolonged PT and PTT to determine the correct treatment, if one is needed. This often requires the determination of selected coagulation factor levels. It is a common mistake to replace factors by infusing the patient with fresh-frozen plasma without identifying the cause of the factor deficiencies and the associated prolongations of the PT and/or PTT.

It is the rare physician who recalls which factors are associated with only a prolonged PTT, only a prolonged PT, or a prolongation of both the PT and the PTT. Generally speaking, the factors associated with a prolonged PTT and a normal PT are the hours in the workday morning, 8 o'clock, 9 o'clock, but not 10 o'clock because it is a coffee break, 11 o'clock, and 12 noon. Thus, deficiencies of factors VIII, IX, XI, and XII are associated with a prolonged PTT in the presence of a normal PT. The factor associated with a prolonged PT in the presence of a normal PTT is factor VII, or the month of July when new residents appear on the staff. The factors in the common pathway of the coagulation cascade, when deficient, most often prolong the PT and the PTT, though the PT is affected more than the PTT. These common pathway factors can be remembered as the smallest denominations of paper currency in the United States; namely, the $1 bill, the $2 bill, the $5 bill, and the $10 bill. Thus, deficiencies of factors I (fibrinogen), II, V, and X commonly prolong both the PT and the PTT.

TEST ORDERING MISTAKES

Ordering the incorrect coagulation factors from lack of knowledge about which coagulation factor deficiencies are associated with a PT prolongation and which coagulation factor deficiencies are associated with a PTT prolongation. For a PTT prolongation with a normal PT value, the most commonly identified factor deficiencies to consider are factors VIII, IX, XI, and XII. For a PT prolongation with a normal PTT value, the most important consideration is a deficiency of factor VII. Deficiencies of fibrinogen (factor I) and factors II, V, and X usually prolong both the PT and PTT. However, mild deficiencies in these factors may prolong only the PT.

▨ *Ordering coagulation factor assays while a patient is receiving warfarin.* Patients receiving warfarin will have deficiencies of factors II, VII, IX, and X, and there is rarely any need to order factor assays to demonstrate these deficiencies in warfarin-treated patients.

▨ *Ordering coagulation factor assays while a patient is receiving a direct thrombin inhibitor, most commonly argatroban.* Thrombin, factor IIa, is near the very bottom of the coagulation cascade. Therefore, for all clot-based assays of coagulation factors, direct thrombin inhibitors will significantly interfere with these tests and provide uninterpretable results for the coagulation factors.

▨ *Confusing factor V with the factor V Leiden mutation.* For patients who are bleeding and being evaluated for a factor V deficiency, the correct test is the factor V assay. For patients who have experienced thrombosis, the correct test is the factor V Leiden.

▨ *Confusing factor II (prothrombin) with the prothrombin 20210 mutation.* For patients who are bleeding and being evaluated for a factor II deficiency, the correct test is the factor II or prothrombin assay. For patients who have experienced thrombosis, the correct test is the assay for the prothrombin 20210 mutation.

▨ *Confusing factor IX with factor XI.* The reversal of the X and the I can result in major errors in treatment that are expensive and can have serious adverse effects. For example, many factor XI–deficient patients need no treatment at all, and factor IX–deficient patients are often given expensive recombinant factor IX concentrate.

▨ *Confusing factor II with factor XI.* It is important to remember that the correct numbering system for coagulation factors involves the use of Roman numerals. If a regular Arabic number (ie, 11) is used to identify the number of the coagulation factor, an assay for factor II is often performed in the clinical laboratory.

MISTAKES IN RESULT INTERPRETATION

■ *Treating all coagulation factor deficiencies with fresh-frozen plasma as a source of the deficient factor.* It should first be understood that not all factor deficiencies are associated with bleeding. Patients with even complete deficiencies of factor XII do not experience bleeding. Many patients with a significant factor VII or factor XI deficiency also do not bleed. The treatment for factor deficiencies depends on the cause and the risk for bleeding. Many physicians incorrectly do not bother to determine if a factor deficiency is a result of an inherited factor deficiency, a result of anticoagulation or a component of a physiologic or pathologic process such as DIC, or a consequence of liver disease. The treatment for a deficiency of the same coagulation factor can be very different in different clinical settings.

■ *Confusing a low level of a PTT-related coagulation factor (factors VIII, IX, XI, and XII) caused by a lupus anticoagulant with a congenital deficiency of one of these four factors.* For example, confusing a patient with a lupus anticoagulant who has low levels of one or more PTT-related coagulation factors with a patient who has factor VIII deficiency can result in the infusion of expensive and potentially prothrombotic coagulation factor concentrates when they are completely unnecessary.

■ *Concluding that slight elevations in the PT or the PTT are always clinically insignificant.* This is a difficult circumstance because in most cases, minor elevations of a few seconds above the upper limit of normal for the PT and the PTT are indeed not often associated with a significant predisposition for bleeding. However, for the patient who has a single factor deficiency, such as a deficiency of factor IX, a persistent slight prolongation of the PTT may be associated with a congenitally low level of factor IX between 20% and 30%. If such a patient is taken to surgery and not provided with factor IX preoperatively, excess bleeding is likely to occur. Therefore, in the absence of a clear explanation for a slight elevation in the PT or the PTT, appropriate factor assays may be informative to identify single congenital factor deficiencies that can predispose the patient to bleeding.

Attempting to completely normalize the PT and the PTT in the patient who has liver disease and concomitantly a deficiency of multiple coagulation factors. In patients with liver disease, slight prolongations of the PT and the PTT are rarely associated with an increased predisposition to bleed. In such patients, attempts to bring the PT and the PTT within the reference range, rather than leaving them slightly above the upper limit of normal, often results in volume overload. If the patient has a prolonged PT and PTT on the basis of liver disease alone, minor elevations in the PT and PTT are often well tolerated. Therefore, it is not appropriate to continue to transfuse fresh-frozen plasma to fully normalize the PT and the PTT in the liver disease patient who is not bleeding.

Failing to understand that the reference ranges for coagulation factors in children may be different from the reference ranges for coagulation factors in adults. For several factors, the reference ranges for children are lower than they are for adults. In addition, the age at which the adult reference range becomes relevant varies with the individual coagulation factor or natural anticoagulant. Because of this, children should be evaluated for deficiencies using the appropriate age-adjusted reference range.

ERRORS WITHIN THE CLINICAL LABORATORY

The clinical laboratory not performing factor assays at multiple plasma dilutions to reveal a factor inhibitor, if it is present. A coagulation factor level may be low because there is decreased synthesis of the factor or because there is an inhibitor of the factor. This differentiation is essential because the treatment for a factor deficiency is usually very different from the treatment for a factor inhibitor. For example, a simple inherited deficiency of factor VIII is often treated with factor VIII concentrate, whereas a deficiency resulting from a clinically apparent factor VIII inhibitor may be treated with recombinant factor VIIa.

■ *The failure to remove heparin, if present, from a plasma specimen before performance of coagulation factor assays and inhibitor testing.* Heparin can be removed from a plasma sample by the addition of a heparin-degrading enzyme to the sample. This will remove the anticoagulant effect of heparin from the sample.

STANDARDS OF CARE

■ Prolongations of the PTT and the PT should lead to the appropriate selection of coagulation factor assays or inhibitors to explain the prolongations identified.

■ Factor inhibitors must be differentiated from factor deficiencies.

■ Reduced levels of coagulation factors produced by argatroban should not be confused with true deficiencies of coagulation factors.

■ The correct numbering terminology for coagulation factor numbers involves the use of Roman numerals.

■ Factor V and prothrombin tests must be carefully differentiated from the assays for factor V Leiden and the prothrombin 20210 mutations, respectively.

■ Treatment of coagulation factor deficiencies should be directed by the cause of the deficiency and not by replacing the deficient coagulation factors with fresh-frozen plasma without determining the cause of the deficiency.

■ Determination of the cause of a slight prolongation of the PT or PTT must be made, which includes consideration of a clinically significant factor deficiency.

■ Age-adjusted reference ranges must be used in the assessment of children for deficiencies of coagulation factors and natural anticoagulants.

■ The coagulation laboratory must clearly differentiate a lupus anticoagulant from PTT-related factor deficiencies.

■ The coagulation laboratory must remove heparin from samples in which it is present when clot-based coagulation and inhibitor assays need to be performed with the samples.

EVALUATION FOR DISSEMINATED INTRAVASCULAR COAGULATION

DIC results from a stimulus that activates coagulation and thereby consumes platelets and coagulation factors in small blood vessels. The depletion of platelets and coagulation factors in capillaries is the reason why DIC is associated with bleeding rather than thrombosis in the vast majority of cases. Despite the fact that DIC is commonly encountered, the diagnosis of this condition can be very challenging. The parameters that change in patients with DIC, including an elevation in the D-dimer, which is of great importance in establishing a diagnosis of DIC, are similarly altered in a variety of other conditions. There is no single test that specifically indicates the presence of DIC. As a further diagnostic complication, the D-dimer assay can be performed by multiple methodologies that have different reference ranges. Some D-dimer tests are more complex to perform than others. For this reason, a single clinical laboratory may offer one method during the day and another method at other times. This can lead to significant confusion among physicians using the laboratory regarding the diagnosis of DIC because it is not always clear which assay was used to quantify the D-dimer. The treatment of a bleeding episode in DIC is replacement therapy with blood products containing the consumed components. Blood products may successfully stop a bleeding episode in a DIC patient, but they may also be ineffective. The inappropriate use of large numbers of blood products to stop a bleeding episode in a patient with an untreatable underlying cause for DIC should be avoided.

TEST ORDERING MISTAKES

Ordering too many tests to establish a diagnosis of DIC. In DIC, there are many changes that can be detected in the blood. For example, complexes of thrombin and antithrombin are formed in DIC. Although assays are available for the measurement of thrombin–antithrombin complexes, these are impractical for performance at all times, even if they are available in the laboratory. A commonly used panel of tests useful for the diagnosis of DIC in a patient with an identified stimulus for DIC includes a platelet count (commonly decreased in acute DIC), a D-dimer assay (typically elevated in DIC), and a PT (usually prolonged in acute DIC). In addition, a peripheral blood smear (for schistocytes) and a fibrinogen test (most commonly serial fibrinogens to show that the fibrinogen value is decreasing) may be informative. The fibrinogen level is increased above normal, as part of the acute-phase response, by many of the stimuli for DIC. This is why a single fibrinogen test that is often normal in DIC can be uninformative. The D-dimer assay provides logistical advantages over the assay for fibrinogen degradation products (FDP), but an elevated FDP result can also be used to provide evidence of clot formation and clot degradation in DIC.

MISTAKES IN RESULT INTERPRETATION

Confusing DIC with liver disease. In both DIC and liver disease, it is not uncommon to find a decreased platelet count, an elevated D-dimer, and an elevated PT. These changes occur by different mechanisms in the two disorders. In the absence of abnormalities in liver function tests, there is minimal difficulty in differentiating DIC from liver disease. However, when liver function tests are clearly abnormal, it may be difficult or impossible to determine if the laboratory changes are attributable to liver disease, DIC, or both. Severe liver failure is a known stimulus for DIC, so the presence of both abnormalities at the same time is a strong possibility.

▨ *Overlooking a diagnosis of compensated DIC.* This can be a challenging diagnosis because, with the exception of an elevated D-dimer or FDP, the other major parameters of the DIC panel can be normal. Increased platelet production in the bone marrow can compensate for a low-grade consumption of platelets in DIC. Similarly, increased synthesis of coagulation factors in the liver can compensate for a low-grade consumption of coagulation factors in DIC. The potential danger of overlooking compensated DIC is that a minor challenge to such a patient, like an infection, can greatly reduce the compensatory actions of the bone marrow and the liver. This will result in the rapid appearance of significantly abnormal values for both the platelet count and the PT. It is reasonable to make the diagnosis of compensated DIC in retrospect, when the compensatory effects are no longer present.

▨ *Unless there are other reasons to do so, treatment of the patient with acute DIC who is not bleeding, using blood products to normalize a low platelet count (with platelet concentrates) or an elevated PT (with fresh-frozen plasma) or a low fibrinogen (with cryoprecipitate).*

▨ *The expectation that it is possible to stop a bleeding episode associated with an underlying DIC stimulus that cannot be effectively treated.* For example, patients with pancreatic cancer who develop DIC are highly unlikely to have the stimulus for DIC removed. On the other hand, a woman with

DIC as a result of a fetal death in utero can rapidly recover from DIC upon delivery of the stillborn fetus. Thoughtful use of blood products is essential in the bleeding patient with DIC because it is possible to greatly deplete the hospital supply of platelet concentrates, fresh-frozen plasma, and cryoprecipitate for a patient with DIC and an untreatable underlying disorder.

OTHER MISTAKES

Clinical laboratories can use a variety of test methodologies for measurement of D-dimer. This test is used in the diagnosis of DIC and to rule out, when negative, venous thrombosis. A negative enzyme-linked immunoassay for D-dimer has long been the gold standard to rule out pulmonary embolism or deep vein thrombosis in the outpatient presenting for evaluation. The most widely used precursor assay of the enzyme-linked D-dimer immunoassay is a latex bead agglutination test. This assay has less sensitivity for the D-dimer than the enzyme-linked immunoassay, but it is extremely easy to perform. Because the enzyme-linked immunoassay is more technically complex, many clinical laboratories offer this higher sensitivity enzyme-linked immunoassay D-dimer measurement during the day, and switch to a latex agglutination test for the evening and night shifts in the laboratory. To add to the confusion, D-dimer assays by different methodologies can have different thresholds to determine when the test is positive. It can be extremely confusing to physicians who use a laboratory with multiple D-dimer assays to know which assay was performed on the samples collected from their patients, and because of this problem, to correctly interpret the test results. At this time, no approach has been widely adopted to address the problem of multiple D-dimer assays, with different levels of technical complexity and different reference ranges. If a clinical laboratory also offers, as part of a DIC panel, assays for FDP by a variety of methodologies, the confusion for physicians with regard to test selection and result interpretation for DIC is even greater.

STANDARDS OF CARE

- The platelet count, the D-dimer, and the PT, with the possible addition of serial fibrinogen testing and a review of a peripheral blood smear, represent an acceptable and widely used group of tests to establish or rule out a diagnosis of DIC.
- Standard liver function tests may be useful to determine if DIC, liver disease, or both are present.
- Compensated DIC should be considered in patients who have a chronic stimulus for DIC, but this diagnosis may only become apparent when the compensatory mechanisms fail.
- Unless there are other reasons to do so, treatment of the acute DIC patient who is not bleeding with blood products is not indicated.
- The continued use of large amounts of blood products in the treatment of the bleeding patient with DIC should be guided by the treatability of the underlying condition stimulating the development of DIC.
- Education of physicians using the clinical laboratory about the assays used for D-dimer and FDP, in particular how they should be used clinically and their diagnostic limitations, is necessary to allow physicians to correctly interpret the results from these assays.

EVALUATION FOR A CONGENITAL HYPERCOAGULABLE STATE

There are several major challenges associated with evaluating a patient for hypercoagulability. One challenge is the identification of appropriate tests for inclusion in the hypercoagulation evaluation. There are five commonly assessed inherited conditions that predispose to thrombosis: the factor V Leiden mutation, the prothrombin 20210 mutation, and deficiencies of protein C, protein S, and antithrombin. Another challenge is to decide which patients should be evaluated with tests for hypercoagulability. There is no consensus on which patients to test even within the United States, and there is substantially more variability when comparing hypercoagulability testing in the United States with hypercoagulation test ordering practices in other countries. Included in the following section are widely recognized errors in test ordering and test result interpretation in the assessment of patients for a congenital hypercoagulable state. Other chapters in this book present information on errors in the evaluation for antiphospholipid antibodies and for HIT that are associated with hypercoagulable states.

TEST ORDERING MISTAKES

- *Ordering protein C and protein S levels in patients being treated with warfarin.* True baseline protein C and protein S levels can be determined reliably two weeks after discontinuation of warfarin therapy, assuming the patient is able to synthesize proteins at a normal rate in the liver.
- *Ordering the clot-based activated protein C resistance assay while the patient has a lupus anticoagulant or is receiving argatroban.* All of these will interfere with this assay. To assess for the presence of factor V Leiden in such cases, the genetic test for the mutation must be performed, and the clot-based test for activated protein C resistance must be omitted.
- *Ordering standard clot-based assays for protein C, protein S, and antithrombin while the patient is receiving argatroban.* These compounds do not interfere with chromogenic assays, such as the chromogenic assay

for protein C. These assays can only be performed if argatroban is no longer present in the specimen.

Ordering an assay for antithrombin for a patient who has been treated with full-dose unfractionated heparin or low molecular weight heparin. With such therapy, antithrombin forms a complex with heparin or low molecular weight heparin that is cleared, resulting in a low level for antithrombin that is not indicative of a true baseline antithrombin level for the patient. The patient's baseline antithrombin can be determined reliably one week after discontinuation of heparin or low molecular weight heparin therapy, assuming the patient is able to synthesize proteins at a normal rate in the liver.

Confusing factor V with the factor V Leiden mutation. For patients who are bleeding and being evaluated for a factor V deficiency, the correct test is the factor V assay. For patients who have experienced thrombosis, the correct test is the factor V Leiden.

Confusing factor II (prothrombin) with the prothrombin 20210 mutation. For patients who are bleeding and being evaluated for a factor II deficiency, the correct test is the factor II or prothrombin assay. For patients who have experienced thrombosis and are being evaluated for thrombotic risk, the correct test is the prothrombin 20210 mutation.

Ordering protein S total antigen instead of protein S free antigen to assess for adequacy of protein S. The protein S total antigen is rarely decreased, and the functional protein S value correlates to the protein S free antigen.

Ordering antigenic tests for protein C, protein S, and antithrombin as first-line assays to assess for deficiencies of these proteins. Functional assays should be the first-line tests, as some patients who have deficiencies in these proteins will have normal antigenic levels but low functional levels. Ordering antigenic tests initially could result in a failure to identify important functional deficiencies of these three proteins.

■ *Ordering the test for methylene tetrahydrofolate reductase (MTHFR) as a risk factor for thrombosis.* There is no proven association between abnormal levels of this enzyme and risk for thrombosis. It was recently thought that an elevated homocysteine is the thrombotic risk factor rather than an alteration in the activity of this enzyme in the homocysteine metabolic pathway. Ultimately, however, homocysteine was also disregarded as a risk factor for thrombosis, at least for modestly elevated homocysteine values that occur with minor vitamin deficiencies and renal dysfunction.

■ *Ordering only protein C, protein S, and antithrombin for the patient to be evaluated for a hypercoagulable state, and omitting the more recently discovered common hypercoagulable states produced by the factor V Leiden mutation and the prothrombin 20210 mutation.*

MISTAKES IN RESULT INTERPRETATION

■ *Concluding that a deficiency of protein C, protein S, and/or antithrombin produced by an acquired condition is associated with an increased thrombotic risk.* For the vast majority of cases, it is the congenital deficiencies of these proteins that result in an increased thrombotic risk. For example, patients with liver disease may demonstrate low levels of protein C, protein S, and antithrombin because these proteins are made in the liver. These patients are, however, typically not at increased risk for thrombosis because liver disease is also associated with deficiencies of the coagulation factors necessary to produce clotting. Therefore, liver disease has an effect that is both prothrombotic and antithrombotic, and as a result, the deficiencies of protein C, protein S, and antithrombin in patients with liver disease are not generally associated with an increased risk for thrombosis. A relatively balanced risk between thrombosis and bleeding is also seen in the patient ingesting warfarin at therapeutic levels.

These patients have a low protein C and a low protein S, but they also have low levels of factors II, VII, IX, and X. The same can also be said for the patient who is being treated with heparin, who experiences a reduced antithrombin level as a result of heparin therapy.

A confusing situation arises for low protein S values associated with two acquired conditions—a high estrogen state and an acute-phase reaction. A low value for protein S is found in patients with increased estrogen, such as those who are pregnant or taking estrogen supplements in the form of oral contraceptives or estrogen replacement therapy. The protein S can also be low in patients experiencing an acute-phase reaction. The high estrogen state and the acute-phase reaction do represent prothrombotic conditions, but the thrombotic tendency is not exclusively associated with the low value for protein S. There are a variety of coagulation abnormalities produced by a high estrogen state or an acute-phase response that promote thrombosis. Therefore, a low protein S associated with pregnancy or estrogen supplementation or an acute-phase response is in itself not considered a single major risk factor for thrombosis.

Failing to understand that the reference ranges for protein C, protein S, and antithrombin in children are different from the corresponding reference ranges for these factors in adults. Protein C is especially late in normalizing to the adult reference range and values for children below the age of eight or nine years are not correctly assessed using the adult reference range. Because of this, children should be evaluated for protein C, protein S, and antithrombin using an appropriate age-adjusted reference range for each factor.

CONTROVERSIES

Ordering protein C, protein S, and antithrombin in patients who are actively clotting. Active clotting is associated with consumption of these factors, and therefore, deficiencies observed during this time do not reflect the patient's true baseline levels of these natural anticoagulant proteins. It is important to not misdiagnose a patient as congenitally deficient in protein C, protein S, or antithrombin during a period of active clotting. Many such patients show only a mild decrease in these three proteins, such that diagnosis of a deficiency state, if one exists, is still usually possible during clot formation. These patients typically increase their levels of these proteins to their baseline values, whatever they are, within a day or two after an acute thrombotic event, assuming normal liver function to permit protein synthesis at a normal rate. Some physicians recommend tests for these proteins only after an acute thrombotic event has clearly subsided, and often when the patient is no longer in the hospital. Other physicians recommend immediate testing so that the patient is sure to be evaluated for a hypercoagulable state. In addition, collection of a blood sample before a patient with venous thrombosis receives anticoagulants provides laboratory values for protein C, protein S, and antithrombin that are not confounded by anticoagulant therapy.

▪ *Considering the homocysteine value to assess for thrombotic risk.* Modest elevations of homocysteine associated with vitamin deficiencies or renal dysfunction do not appear to be associated with an increased thrombotic risk. However, it has not been established whether very significantly elevated homocysteine values, for example, above 30 µmol/L, are associated with thrombotic risk. Patients with very high homocysteine levels may have an inherited defect in homocysteine metabolism. One congenital disorder associated with markedly elevated homocysteine levels is a deficiency of the enzyme cystathionine beta-synthase.

▪ *Ordering hypercoagulation studies prior to making a decision about the use of oral contraceptives.* The combination of oral contraceptives and a genetic deficiency associated with thrombosis greatly increases the risk of a clotting event. For that reason, some argue that a hypercoagulation panel should be performed before prescribing oral contraceptives. The cost to the health care system from evaluating women with a negative personal and family thrombotic history with hypercoagulation studies is not insignificant, and this is the principal argument for not performing the tests. At a minimum, however, there is wide agreement that a careful personal history and family history for thrombosis should be taken before providing any recommendation for oral contraceptive use.

STANDARDS OF CARE

- Order tests for activated protein C resistance, protein C, protein S, and antithrombin in the absence of interfering factors, commonly anticoagulants, which make the results of these tests uninterpretable and not representative of the patient's true baseline values.
- Order functional rather than antigenic tests for protein C, protein S, and antithrombin as first-line tests for assessment of hypercoagulability.
- Avoid the use of MTHFR as a test for thrombotic risk, and do not conclude that modest elevations in homocysteine represent a risk for thrombosis.
- Identify the factor V Leiden mutation and the prothrombin 20210 mutation and congenital deficiencies of protein C, protein S, and antithrombin as risks for thrombosis, with the understanding that acquired deficiencies of protein C, protein S, and antithrombin are unlikely to represent risks for thrombosis because these deficiencies typically occur at the same time when there is an increased risk for bleeding.
- Age-adjusted reference ranges must be used in the assessment of children for deficiencies of protein C, protein S, and antithrombin.

EVALUATION FOR ANTIPHOSPHOLIPID ANTIBODIES

For patients with thrombotic disorders, tests for antiphospholipid antibodies are commonly performed. Antiphospholipid antibodies represent a large category of antibodies directed at the protein beta-2 glycoprotein I. The function of this protein and its relationship to thrombosis remain to be fully elucidated, although much progress is being made. Antibodies to beta-2 glycoprotein I can be measured in a clot-based assay known as the lupus anticoagulant test. In addition, such antibodies can be detected in enzyme-linked immunoassay tests for anticardiolipin antibodies and for anti–beta-2 glycoprotein I antibodies, and these may be specific to domain 1 of the beta-2 glycoprotein I protein. There is another increasingly recognized antiphospholipid antibody that recognizes factor II (prothrombin), which is bound to the negatively charged phospholipid known as phosphatidylserine. There is substantial confusion among practitioners regarding which antiphospholipid antibody tests should be ordered and how the results for these tests should be interpreted. In general, the more of the antiphospholipid antibody tests that are positive, and the higher the test results are above the upper limit of normal, the greater is the risk for a thrombotic event.

TEST ORDERING MISTAKES

Failing to order enough tests to assess for antiphospholipid antibodies. There is a growing consensus that, among the different antiphospholipid antibody tests, the lupus anticoagulant test is the one most associated with thrombotic risk. However, some patients have a negative test for the lupus anticoagulant, while testing positive for anticardiolipin antibodies or anti–beta-2 glycoprotein I antibodies. For this reason, if a patient is being evaluated for thrombotic risk with tests for antiphospholipid antibodies, tests for the lupus anticoagulant as well as tests for anticardiolipin or anti–beta-2 glycoprotein I antibodies should be performed to complete a thorough evaluation for the presence of an antiphospholipid antibody.

■ *Ordering too many antiphospholipid antibody tests.* There are many tests commercially available for the lupus anticoagulant. A screening test and a confirmatory test that are phospholipid dependent have long been considered adequate to assess a patient or the lupus anticoagulant. There are at least five other commercially available tests for the lupus anticoagulant. For anticardiolipin antibodies, it is possible to test for IgG, IgM, and IgA antibodies. The same three antibody classes can also be measured for anti–beta-2 glycoprotein I antibodies. There are also commercially available tests for anti-prothrombin and antiphosphatidylserine antibodies (IgG, IgM, and IgA). A common practice is to quantify only IgG and IgM antibodies when assessing a patient for anticardiolipin antibodies or anti–beta-2 glycoprotein I antibodies. Thus, one can perform more than a dozen different tests to search for antiphospholipid antibodies, but performing these tests until one is found to be positive is considered inappropriate.

■ *Not performing a confirmatory phospholipid-dependent test for the lupus anticoagulant following a positive screening test.* Screening tests for the lupus anticoagulant based on the PTT have many interferences that generate false-positive test results. For this reason, a confirmatory phospholipid-dependent assay for the lupus anticoagulant is essential to accurately determine whether the patient has a lupus anticoagulant.

MISTAKES IN RESULT INTERPRETATION

■ *Concluding that the presence of a lupus anticoagulant is an indication that the patient has the disease systemic lupus erythematosus or that the patient has an anticoagulant.* Unfortunately, the lupus anticoagulant was first found in two women with lupus and was named as a result of this association. Many healthy asymptomatic individuals and many patients with disorders other than autoimmune diseases are found to have a lupus anticoagulant. Also unfortunately, the lupus anticoagulant was found to prolong the time for clot formation in laboratory coagulation tests. Paradoxically, in vivo, the presence of the lupus anticoagulant itself does not confer a bleeding risk, but may confer a thrombotic risk. Thus, both "lupus" and "anticoagulant" are misleading terms.

▦ *Confusing a lupus anticoagulant for a factor VIII inhibitor and confusing a factor VIII inhibitor for a lupus anticoagulant.* It is often difficult to conclusively demonstrate that a patient has one of these entities but not the other. Clinically, however, it is extremely important to do so, because patients with a factor VIII inhibitor may have catastrophic bleeding, and patients with the lupus anticoagulant may develop serious thrombosis. As a result, the treatment for these two entities is completely the opposite. The challenge arises because the presence of a factor VIII inhibitor can produce a false-positive test for the lupus anticoagulant; and the presence of a lupus anticoagulant can result in a low factor VIII level in the test for coagulation factor VIII in the laboratory. One way to attempt to differentiate a lupus anticoagulant from a factor VIII inhibitor is to perform assays for coagulation factors VIII, IX, XI, and XII. These are all PTT-related coagulation factor assays, and as noted previously, the lupus anticoagulant in the vast majority of cases prolongs the PTT and not the PT. The assays for coagulation factors should be performed at multiple plasma dilutions to assess for the presence of a coagulation factor inhibitor. When a lupus anticoagulant is present, an inhibitor is detected in more than one of the four PTT-related coagulation factor assays, and the factors that are lowered are decreased approximately to the same extent by this inhibitor. On the other hand, factor VIII inhibitors typically result in a markedly low value only for factor VIII, with higher values for factors IX, XI, and XII. Some patients with a factor VIII inhibitor will have a negative test for a lupus anticoagulant. When this situation arises, it is much easier to differentiate the patient with a factor VIII inhibitor from one with the lupus anticoagulant.

CONTROVERSIES

▓ *It is still not well established whether it is advisable to evaluate a patient for antiphospholipid antibodies using both anticardiolipin antibody tests and anti–beta-2 glycoprotein I antibody tests.* These are both enzyme-linked immunoassay tests in which an antibody from the patient binds to the protein beta-2 glycoprotein I. The assays are constructed somewhat differently, and for that reason there is a concern that an antibody might be detected using one assay but not the other. Generally speaking, if there is a high suspicion for an antiphospholipid antibody in a patient with a negative test for the lupus anticoagulant, tests for anticardiolipin antibodies and anti–beta-2 glycoprotein I antibodies might both be ordered in an effort to detect antiphospholipid antibodies. Enthusiasm is decreasing at the present time for the use of anticardiolipin antibody tests.

STANDARDS OF CARE

▓ The assessment of a patient for the presence of antiphospholipid antibodies should include a correctly performed screening test and a phospholipid-dependent lupus anticoagulant test if the screening test is positive, as well as assays for IgG and

IgM anticardiolipin or anti–beta-2 glycoprotein I antibodies.

A lupus anticoagulant must be clearly differentiated from a factor VIII inhibitor.

Patients with a lupus anticoagulant alone should not be presumed to have the disease lupus or to suffer from a bleeding predisposition.

EVALUATION FOR VON WILLEBRAND DISEASE

The diagnosis of von Willebrand disease is typically initiated with a request for tests for von Willebrand factor antigen, ristocetin cofactor, and factor VIII. Patients can significantly elevate their values for these assays above their true baseline levels with even a mild stimulation of the acute-phase response. As a result, many patients who have a von Willebrand factor level or ristocetin cofactor level consistent with von Willebrand disease are misdiagnosed as being free from the disease because their values were elevated as part of the acute-phase response at the time they were studied. Repeat testing in the absence of all stimuli to the acute-phase response is absolutely essential, and this may require several evaluations of the patient to confidently determine whether a patient has von Willebrand disease.

TEST ORDERING MISTAKES

Ordering a von Willebrand multimer analysis to further evaluate a patient whose results for von Willebrand factor antigen, ristocetin cofactor, and factor VIII strongly indicate the presence of type 1 von Willebrand disease. Most patients with von Willebrand disease have type 1. Therefore, unless there is a reason from the results of the initial tests for von Willebrand factor, ristocetin cofactor, and factor VIII to suspect a von

Willebrand type other than type 1, it is unnecessary to test for von Willebrand multimers.

Not ordering a complete von Willebrand panel, which minimally consists of tests for von Willebrand factor antigen and ristocetin cofactor. The inclusion of factor VIII is often informative and considered necessary by many in the initial screening for von Willebrand disease. The test for ristocetin cofactor shows much analytical variability and is time-consuming. Because of this, for cases requiring a rapid indication of the presence or absence of von Willebrand disease, a von Willebrand factor antigen test may be useful as an initial assessment of the disease. However, final conclusions regarding a diagnosis of von Willebrand disease should be made using the results from von Willebrand factor antigen and ristocetin cofactor, and factor VIII if it is performed.

MISTAKES IN RESULT INTERPRETATION

Failing to understand that von Willebrand factor, as measured by von Willebrand factor antigen and as ristocetin cofactor, increases in the presence of an acute-phase response. Therefore, patients suffering from infections, patients who have been injured, and those affected by other stimuli of the acute-phase response can experience an increase of 2- to 3-fold over baseline of both von Willebrand factor antigen and ristocetin cofactor. This can result in the incorrect conclusion that a patient with a von Willebrand factor baseline level well below normal is completely free of von Willebrand disease.

Failing to understand that the reference range for von Willebrand factor antigen in children less than six months of age is higher than the reference range for this protein in individuals older than six months. Therefore, a value that might be normal for someone older than six months could be low for a child younger than six months. Because of this, children should be evaluated for von Willebrand disease using an appropriate age-adjusted reference range.

CONTROVERSIES

The threshold for von Willebrand factor antigen and ristocetin cofactor, below which a diagnosis of von Willebrand disease is rendered, remains controversial. The trend has been to use increasingly lower thresholds to establish the diagnosis of this disease. Guidelines driven by opinion experts are emerging, but there is significant controversy about them because so many patients above a threshold recommended for diagnosis of von Willebrand disease clearly have a bleeding disorder that is decreased by elevation of von Willebrand factor with DDAVP. These patients do not formally qualify for a diagnosis.

A major confounding variable in the establishment of a reference range for von Willebrand disease using von Willebrand factor or ristocetin cofactor is that the blood type of the patient greatly influences the amount of von Willebrand factor. Patients with blood group O have approximately 74% of the normal amount of von Willebrand factor, and patients with type AB blood have as much as 125% of the normal amount of von Willebrand factor. Patients with type A or type B have mean values between 74% and 125%, with type B patients being higher than patients with type A. The general consensus at this point appears to consider bleeding risk based on the absolute amount of von Willebrand factor and ristocetin cofactor, independent of the blood type. As a result, patients with type O blood require a modest decrease in von Willebrand factor or ristocetin cofactor from their mean value of 74% to receive a diagnosis of von Willebrand disease. This is in contrast to the patient with type AB blood who requires a major decrease from 125% to achieve a diagnosis of von Willebrand disease.

STANDARDS OF CARE

▨ The appropriate testing to initially evaluate a patient for von Willebrand disease includes von Willebrand factor antigen and ristocetin cofactor minimally, with factor VIII commonly included in the initial testing.

▨ Normal values for von Willebrand factor antigen and ristocetin cofactor in a bleeding patient suspected of von Willebrand disease should be considered as possibly elevated from an acute-phase stimulus. Repeat testing for the disease should be performed to confirm or deny the presence of this disorder if there is reason to be suspicious of an acute phase response.

▨ Despite variations in von Willebrand factor antigen and ristocetin cofactor with blood type, the threshold for diagnosis of von Willebrand disease is commonly made without consideration of the patient's blood type.

▨ Age-adjusted reference ranges must be used in the diagnosis of von Willebrand disease.

EVALUATION FOR A COAGULATION FACTOR VIII INHIBITOR

The presence of a factor VIII inhibitor can lead to major bleeding. The identification of the inhibitor, which requires its differentiation from the lupus anticoagulant and its subsequent quantitation in Bethesda units, is essential to identifying and correctly managing the patient with a factor VIII inhibitor. The test for the factor VIII inhibitor is one of the most complex assays performed in the clinical laboratory. It should be performed only in cases in which there is significant evidence from a PTT mixing study and a factor VIII assay (as detailed under Test Ordering Mistakes which follows) that a factor VIII inhibitor is present. The treatment options for a factor VIII inhibitor are all extremely expensive (cases have been reported in which hundreds of thousands of dollars have been spent on a single patient), and they all present a measurable thrombotic risk. Thus, it is possible to convert a bleeding patient with a factor VIII inhibitor into one with a catastrophic thrombosis. The treatment selected is significantly influenced by the Bethesda unit value. Therefore, the accurate measurement of antibodies to factor VIII is important because it guides the appropriate use of highly expensive and potentially thrombotic compounds.

TEST ORDERING MISTAKES

Requesting quantitation of the antibody to factor VIII in Bethesda units when there is no evidence from the PTT mixing study or the factor VIII level to suspect an antibody to factor VIII. The PTT mixing study shows a classic response in patients with a factor VIII inhibitor. The PTT of the mixed plasma initially corrects into the reference range or shortens significantly toward normal, but as the mixed plasma is allowed to incubate at 37°C for up to 1 to 2 hours, the PTT increases. The antibody to factor VIII requires time in the mixed plasma to bind and neutralize the factor VIII, and thereby produce this result in the mixing study (initial correction which fades) suggestive of a factor VIII inhibitor. The PTT increase over the incubation time in the mixing study with normal plasma is approximately reflective of the strength of the inhibitor in Bethesda units.

MISTAKES IN RESULT INTERPRETATION

Incorrectly identifying a lupus anticoagulant, present in 3% to 5% of healthy individuals, as a much rarer factor VIII inhibitor, and conversely mistaking a rare factor VIII inhibitor as a lupus anticoagulant. This situation is presented in significant detail on pages 102–103 on antiphospholipid antibodies under the "Mistakes in Result Interpretation" section.

▓ *Treating a patient with a factor VIII inhibitor with factor VIII concentrate when the Bethesda unit level indicates that there is too much anti–factor VIII antibody for the concentrate to be effective.* Bethesda unit values above 4 to 10 (published studies show different thresholds within this range) should indicate a need to use a product other than factor VIII concentrate to treat bleeding. Commonly used treatments for such patients include recombinant factor VIIa and prothrombin complex concentrates. It is useful to note that in most patients with a factor VIII inhibitor, each additional Bethesda unit decreases the amount of factor VIII by approximately 50%. Therefore, only seven Bethesda units can decrease a value of 100% factor VIII to: 50% (1), 25% (2), 12.5% (3), 6.25% (4), 3.12% (5), 1.66% (6), and 0.8% (7). Many patients with factor VIII inhibitors have values above seven Bethesda units.

STANDARDS OF CARE

▓ The highly complex and expensive test for quantitation of the antibody to factor VIII in Bethesda units should not be ordered unless there is evidence from the PTT mixing study or the factor VIII level to suspect an antibody to factor VIII.

▓ A factor VIII inhibitor and a lupus anticoagulant should be clearly differentiated, using the appropriate laboratory tests.

▓ The treatment option selected for a patient with a factor VIII inhibitor should be appropriate for the number of Bethesda units quantitated in the assay.

EVALUATION FOR THROMBOCYTOPENIA THAT IS NOT ASSOCIATED WITH HEPARIN EXPOSURE

Errors associated with spuriously high or low platelet counts are commonly observed in the clinical laboratory. One of the most common causes of a spuriously low platelet count results from a problem of insufficient mixing at the time of blood collection. This can occur when the blood in the tube is not gently agitated back and forth several times to mix the dried EDTA anticoagulant in the tube with the blood. In some cases, the laboratory can identify a platelet count as spurious by further analysis before it is reported. However, in other situations, the physician needs to have a high level of suspicion that a platelet count, which is significantly different from recent platelet counts on the same patient, is spurious, to avoid a misdiagnosis. Laboratory testing can be performed to identify a limited number of causes for a true thrombocytopenia. Such laboratory tests, however, are often present only in large clinical laboratories. Examples of these assays are the ADAMTS 13 assays for thrombotic thrombocytopenic purpura (TTP) and drug-induced thrombocytopenia assays for heparin and compounds other than heparin.

TEST ORDERING MISTAKES

- *Not considering a medication recently initiated for a patient as a cause for thrombocytopenia.* There are many medications that are associated with the development of thrombocytopenia. Although uncommonly performed, assays are available to assess for drug-induced thrombocytopenia for compounds other than heparin. A positive test in such an assay provides at least a tentative diagnosis for drug-induced thrombocytopenia associated with that drug. A confirmed diagnosis can be established if the platelet count recovers after discontinuation of the suspected medication.

■ *Ordering a test for antiplatelet antibodies by flow cytometry or other method in the diagnostic evaluation for immune thrombocytopenia (ITP).* Although such testing is available, it has minimal clinical utility in this setting.

MISTAKES IN RESULT INTERPRETATION

■ *Overlooking platelet clumping induced by EDTA in a purple top Vacutainer containing EDTA as an anticoagulant.* Such platelet clumping leads to a diagnosis of "pseudo-thrombocytopenia" because the platelet count is not decreased in the patient, only in the blood sample. A review of a blood smear made with a sample of whole blood from such a patient would reveal platelet clumps to suggest a diagnosis of pseudo-thrombocytopenia. Collection of blood for a platelet count into a tube with citrate and no EDTA confirms the diagnosis if the platelet count is normal.

■ *Failing to review and act upon an extremely low platelet count in a timely fashion.* Platelet counts that are especially low, particularly those less than 10,000 per microliter, can be associated with spontaneous bleeding and produce significantly adverse clinical outcomes. A very low platelet count is typically regarded as a critical value requiring immediate notification of a caregiver.

■ *Failing to recognize a low platelet count as attributable to TTP as a possible diagnosis.* TTP is a rare but life-threatening condition. If a patient suffering from TTP is treated by apheresis, the mortality from this disorder decreases dramatically. A constellation of laboratory and clinical findings provides a relative likelihood for a diagnosis of TTP. At the current time, assays for the enzyme activity (ADAMTS 13) deficient in patients with TTP are being performed in a limited number of clinical laboratories. Despite the low incidence of this disorder, the potentially devastating clinical consequences of a missed diagnosis of TTP and the expense and invasiveness of apheresis have all promoted the rapid development of ADAMTS 13 assays that can be performed without especially sophisticated laboratory equipment.

Assuming that thrombocytopenia from all causes is effectively treated with transfusion of platelet concentrates. Platelet transfusions given to patients with this disorder, for example, can result in thrombosis that is associated with significant morbidity and mortality.

OTHER MISTAKES

The failure of the laboratory to recognize platelet clumps, or clots containing platelets, in the collection tube as a result of inadequate sample mixing with the anticoagulant in the tube at the time of collection, when it is possible to do so. In many cases, the platelet clumps are too small to be recognized visually by the technologist in the laboratory. Platelet clumping in the collection tube can significantly lower than the platelet count when it is quantitated in a cell counter. In such cases, it may be difficult for a treating physician to know that a low platelet count is artifactual and that it is decreased as a result of inadequate mixing of blood and anticoagulant by the person collecting the blood sample. Comparing platelet counts over time, if they are available, can raise the suspicion that a single low platelet count is spurious and not reflective of the patient's true condition.

Mistaking particulate matter or microorganisms for platelets in a blood sample analyzed in an automated blood cell counter. In some cases, a presumably high platelet count can be further evaluated immediately in the laboratory by review of the raw data from the cell counter to show that particles or microorganisms roughly the same size and density of platelets are being mistaken as platelets. In other cases, however, when it is impossible for the laboratory to convincingly demonstrate that an artifactually high platelet count is spurious, the physician needs to be suspicious that an elevated platelet count is not truly present.

STANDARDS OF CARE

- The platelet count should be monitored in patients being treated with medications that can lead to thrombocytopenia. The prototype drug in this category is heparin, but other pharmaceutical compounds can also lead to drug-induced thrombocytopenia.
- Platelet clumping induced by EDTA in a purple top collection tube containing EDTA as an anticoagulant should be an early consideration in a patient with a low platelet count and no other obvious explanation.
- Extremely low platelet counts, especially those below 10,000 per microliter, represent critical values and require immediate attention.
- TTP should be considered as a possible diagnosis when thrombocytopenia and the appropriate constellation of clinical and laboratory parameters are present. Prompt institution of apheresis for cases with a high likelihood for TTP is essential.
- Platelet concentrates are not indicated as a treatment for thrombocytopenia from all causes. In fact, platelet concentrates may be contraindicated for certain causes of thrombocytopenia, such as HIT.
- The laboratory should attempt to recognize platelet clumps in the collection tube as a result of inadequate sample mixing with the anticoagulant in the tube at the time of collection, realizing that this is possible only if the clumps are large.

EVALUATION FOR PLATELET DYSFUNCTION IN THE PRESENCE OR ABSENCE OF ANTIPLATELET AGENTS

Assessment of platelet function in clinical laboratories has been performed for many decades using platelet-rich plasma and an assortment of platelet agonists, including collagen, arachidonate, ADP, epinephrine, and ristocetin. Performance of this test is associated with many potential analytical errors that must be avoided to provide the most interpretable result for platelet function. Platelet function can also be assessed using whole blood, with the determination of both platelet aggregation and platelet granule release. Markedly abnormal responses to multiple agonists are likely to indicate abnormal platelet function in vivo. However, predictability of bleeding risk in a patient with minor reductions in platelet activity, particularly with a weak platelet agonist like epinephrine, is highly uncertain.

Recently, new assays have been introduced to offer an assessment of platelets for aspirin and clopidogrel (Plavix) resistance. Platelet function can now be evaluated using several different methodologies. Platelet aggregation is now performed not only to assess baseline platelet function but also to determine if an antiplatelet medication has produced the desired platelet inhibition. In this situation, a desired response is often poor platelet function because it implies that the antiplatelet medication is effective.

TEST ORDERING MISTAKES

Performing tests for baseline platelet function, when the patient has purposely or inadvertently ingested aspirin or other antiplatelet medication before testing. Aspirin is included in a number of over-the-counter preparations that do not have the word aspirin in the name. In addition, a number of aspirin preparations have names that do not suggest that the pill or capsule is indeed aspirin. Because of this, patients can inadvertently ingest aspirin and report no aspirin ingestion. In this situation, platelet dysfunction will be observed as a result of the antiplatelet medication and obscure any endogenous abnormalities that might be present and detectable. If aspirin has been avoided for five to seven days, most of the decreased platelet function should be restored. If aspirin has been avoided for 10 to 14 days, in the absence of other variables, platelet function should be fully restored. Recent ingestion of clopidogrel will also result in abnormal platelet function if the patient effectively converts the oral prodrug into the active antiplatelet medication. Platelet function returns to normal approximately seven days after the last dose of clopidogrel.

■ *Use of the template bleeding time to assess platelet function*. This test is associated with many variables, and currently, it is rarely used to assess the adequacy of platelet function. In particular, it has been shown to be a poorly predictive test for platelet function in the patient anticipating surgery.

MISTAKES IN RESULT INTERPRETATION

■ *Concluding that any reduction in platelet function is associated with an increased risk for bleeding*. In a standard platelet-rich plasma–based platelet aggregation study, for example, the clinical significance of a mildly decreased response to epinephrine is highly uncertain. Minor abnormalities may or may not be associated with an increased risk for bleeding.

■ *Failing to consider the potential antiplatelet effect of medications taken by a patient being evaluated for platelet function*. A careful review of the adverse effect of many pharmaceutical compounds, as well as herbal medicines, indicates that an impairment in platelet function can occur in some percentage of patients taking these drugs. If possible, repeat testing for platelet function in the absence of a drug suspected to be responsible for platelet dysfunction is likely to be informative.

OTHER MISTAKES

The failure of the laboratory to appropriately perform the test for platelet aggregation using platelet-rich plasma. Technical variables that can produce false results (positive or negative) include the following: allowing the sample of platelet-rich plasma to sit too long before a platelet agonist is added; cooling the platelet-rich plasma before the addition of the platelet agonist; addition of the platelet agonist to the wall of the tube containing platelet-rich plasma in such a way that the agonist never fully mixes with the platelet suspension; contamination of the platelet-rich plasma with red blood cells that do not clump in the presence of the platelet agonist and obscure the platelet response; and not assessing the activity of platelet agonists with normal donor platelets as controls when the platelet aggregation responses of the patient are reduced.

CONTROVERSIES

There is growing evidence to support the use of pharmacogenomic testing for CYP2C19. This cytochrome system metabolizes clopidogrel from an oral prodrug to an active platelet antagonist. Patients with decreased function of CYP2C19 are poor responders to clopidogrel and suffer an increased frequency of thrombotic events.

A particularly significant controversy relates to the concept of aspirin sensitivity testing. There are several diagnostic platforms in use to assess the sensitivity of platelets to aspirin. The lack of a consensus-driven guideline for aspirin resistance testing is explained by several factors. One is that a single sample of platelets tested on the multiple available diagnostic platforms for aspirin sensitivity is likely to produce mixed results, with some assays suggesting that a patient's platelets are aspirin sensitive and other assays suggesting that the platelets are aspirin resistant. It is impossible to know which test result reflects the true response of the platelets to aspirin in vivo. A second factor is that there is no universally accepted definition of aspirin resistance. A third issue is that apparent aspirin resistance in many patients taking 81 mg of aspirin daily is overcome by simply increasing the dose to 325 mg daily. These patients appear to be aspirin resistant only at a lower aspirin dose. There is one circumstance that has been widely accepted to produce aspirin resistance. It has been shown that ingestion of a nonsteroidal anti-inflammatory drug, such as ibuprofen, shortly preceding aspirin ingestion can prevent the permanent antiplatelet effect induced by aspirin. Platelets can recover adequate function after exposure to a nonsteroidal anti-inflammatory drug, usually within 24 hours after the drug has been taken. Therefore, aspirin-treated platelets that have been previously exposed to a nonsteroidal anti-inflammatory drug are commonly found to be aspirin resistant because they recover platelet function after exposure to aspirin.

STANDARDS OF CARE

▪ When performing a test for platelet function to assess bleeding risk in the absence of antiplatelet medications, it is necessary for the patient to have avoided aspirin and clopidogrel for, ideally, at least 7 to 10 days before testing. Nonsteroidal anti-inflammatory drugs (NSAIDs) should be avoided for at least 24 hours.

░ It is necessary to take a complete history of prescription and nonprescription medications before platelet function testing, to accurately determine if any platelet function defect is a result of inadvertent ingestion of an antiplatelet medication, most commonly aspirin.

░ Use of the template bleeding time to assess platelet function has been widely abandoned and should not be used to evaluate bleeding risk.

░ A mild reduction in platelet aggregation, as an isolated laboratory finding, should not be considered as a definite risk factor for bleeding.

░ The potential antiplatelet effect of all medications, not just known antiplatelet drugs, being taken by a patient who is evaluated for platelet function must always be considered in the interpretation of platelet function tests.

░ The clinical laboratory must meticulously perform the test for platelet aggregation using platelet-rich plasma to avoid introducing technical variables that can produce false results.

BIBLIOGRAPHY

The following annotated references may be useful in identifying the primary literature for information connected to the standards of care in this chapter.

Colman RW, Hirsh J, Marder VJ, et al, eds. *Hemostasis and Thrombosis, Basic Principles and Clinical Practice.* 5th ed. Philadelphia, PA: Lippincott Williams & Wilkins; 2007.

Hillyer CD, Shaz BH, Zimring JC, eds. Part II: coagulation. In: *Transfusion Medicine and Hemostasis: Clinical and Laboratory Aspects.* Oxford, UK: Elsevier; 2009:433–750.

Marques MB, Fritsma GA. *Coagulation Testing.* 2nd ed. Washington, DC: AACC Press; 2009.

Michelson AD, ed. *Platelets.* 2nd ed. Oxford, UK: Academic Press; 2007.

Van Cott EM, Laposata M. Coagulation. In: Jacobs DS, DeMott WR, Oxley DK, eds. *Jacobs and DeMott Laboratory*

Test Handbook with Key Word Index. 5th ed. Hudson, OH: Lexi-Comp; 2001:327–358.

Van Cott EM, Laposata M. Bleeding and thrombotic disorders. In: Laposata M, ed. *Laboratory Medicine: The Diagnosis of Disease in the Clinical Laboratory*. New York, NY: McGraw-Hill; 2010:chap 11, 235–270.

CHAPTER 3
Hematology and Immunology

ADAM C. SEEGMILLER
MARY ANN THOMPSON ARILDSEN

HEMATOLOGY

PREANALYTICAL ERRORS

Improper collection and/or handling can lead to significant errors in hematology results. Hematology tests are sensitive to errors in specimen collection and handling. Samples collected for complete blood counts (CBCs) and peripheral blood smears should be collected from a peripheral vein, when possible, and transferred into an ethylenediaminetetraacetic acid (EDTA; lavender top) tube, following standard collection protocols, and processed in a timely fashion.

STANDARDS OF CARE

- Two patient identifiers should be confirmed before phlebotomy to ensure that the blood is being drawn from the correct patient. Tubes should be promptly labeled before drawing blood from a subsequent patient. Delta checks should be used in the laboratory to identify potential patient identification errors.

■ For CBC testing, blood should be drawn into an EDTA (lavender top) tube. The tube must be completely filled to ensure that the EDTA concentration is within normal limits. The blood should be well mixed after collection into the tube to prevent clot formation and transported to the laboratory in a timely fashion.

■ If a patient is receiving intravenous fluids, blood samples should be drawn from the opposite arm and from a peripheral vein, whenever possible. If the same arm must be used, the blood should be drawn from a site distal to the intravenous line insertion site.

■ Specimens sent for CBC measurements should be carefully scrutinized in the laboratory for visual changes. They should be rejected if there are visible clots or if there is discernible hemolysis or lipemia.

■ The quality of a peripheral blood smear should be taken into consideration when evaluating blood cell morphology. Smears that are too thick, poorly smeared, or air dried can have red cell artifacts. These possibilities should be considered before reporting significant abnormalities in red blood cell (RBC) morphology.

HEMATOLOGY: RED BLOOD CELLS

ERRORS IN THE EVALUATION OF RBC MORPHOLOGY

RBC morphology, although very useful diagnostically, should not be relied on as a sole diagnostic indicator for any condition. RBCs have a biconcave shape that leads to a typical appearance on peripheral blood smear examination—round cells with central clearing or pallor that occupies approximately one third of the cell diameter. Variations in the shape of RBCs, so-called poikilocytosis, can occur in a number of clinical conditions, and, therefore, review of RBC morphology is an important diagnostic procedure. Many RBC morphology changes can be nonspecific, and their diagnostic value is dependent on the quality of the peripheral smear.

STANDARDS OF CARE

- Peripheral blood smears should be made by an automated slide maker stainer, if possible, to ensure that smears are consistently well made and stained.
- If smears must be prepared manually, the persons preparing the smears should be subjected to rigorous training and appropriate quality control should be performed, because the ability to interpret the smear depends on its quality.
- Specific red cell morphologies should be reported as present using strict and specific criteria. For example, schistocytes should have sharp edges and angles with no central pallor, and target cells and echinocytes should be widely distributed on the smears rather than concentrated on a single part of the smear.

ERRORS IN THE DIAGNOSIS OF ANEMIA

One RBC disorder may be masked by the presence of another leading to misdiagnosis. Anemia is indicated by low hemoglobin and/or hematocrit and is categorized by mean cell volume (MCV) as microcytic, normocytic, or macrocytic. Distinguishing among causes of microcytic anemia is a common clinical problem. The differential diagnosis of microcytic anemia includes iron deficiency, anemia of chronic disease, and selected hemoglobinopathies, including thalassemia. These diagnoses can often be distinguished by a careful examination of the peripheral blood smear and examination of other RBC indices, including the RBC count, red cell distribution width (RDW), and reticulocyte hemoglobin (RetHe), among others. Diagnosis of iron deficiency anemia requires iron studies, including serum iron, total iron-binding capacity (TIBC), transferrin saturation (TSAT), and ferritin, the last of which is the most sensitive indicator. Distinguishing the causes of microcytic anemia can be complicated when there are two or more different disorders at the same time, often leading to incorrect diagnoses.

STANDARDS OF CARE

▦ The diagnosis of microcytic anemia should always include careful inspection of the peripheral blood smear and RBC indices, particularly the Mentzer index (MCV/RBC) to determine if thalassemia or other hemoglobinopathy should be considered in the differential diagnosis.

▦ Complete iron studies, including serum iron, TIBC, TSAT, and ferritin, should always be performed to confirm a presumptive diagnosis of iron deficiency as well as to establish a baseline for determining the efficacy of oral iron therapy. Although ferritin is the most sensitive indicator of iron deficiency, one should not rely on ferritin alone, as it can be falsely elevated in inflammatory states. RetHe should be reviewed when it is difficult to distinguish between iron deficiency and anemia of chronic disease.

▦ If microcytic anemia persists after appropriate oral iron supplementation, the patient should be screened for a hemoglobinopathy. This is especially important in immigrants from areas with a high incidence of hemoglobin mutations who may not have received newborn screening for these disorders.

▦ If hemoglobin S is less than 33% in a patient with sickle cell trait, a search for an additional cause of anemia, such as iron deficiency or alpha-thalassemia, must be initiated.

▦ In a patient with anemia and high suspicion of nutritional deficiency, a normal MCV should prompt examination of iron, vitamin B_{12}, and folate studies to rule out combined deficiencies of these dietary components.

ERRORS IN INTERPRETATION OF RETICULOCYTE COUNT

Potential errors in interpreting reticulocyte counts. Reticulocytes are immature anucleate RBCs that circulate in the peripheral blood. The number of circulating reticulocytes is indicative of underlying erythropoiesis; that is, when erythropoiesis is stimulated, the number of circulating reticulocytes increases. Thus, the reticulocyte count can be used to differentiate anemias that are a result of RBC loss or destruction from anemias that are due to failure of marrow erythropoiesis.

STANDARD OF CARE

■ Absolute reticulocyte counts are preferable to reticulocyte percentages, when they are available. If percentages are used, they should be corrected for the degree of anemia, using the equation for the corrected reticulocyte count.

HEMATOLOGY: WHITE BLOOD CELLS

ERRORS IN THE EVALUATION OF GRANULOCYTIC LEUKOCYTOSIS

Failure to take care to recognize the features of granulocytic leukocytosis, resulting in an incorrect diagnosis and/or an inappropriate therapy. Granulocytic leukocytosis is an abnormality characterized by an elevated white blood cell (WBC) count in which the increase is predominantly due to increased granulocytes. These are usually neutrophils and precursors, but increased eosinophils may also be present. These findings may be accompanied by a "left shift," an increase in circulating neutrophil precursors, such as bands and metamyelocytes. Marked granulocytic leukocytosis with a left shift is often called a leukemoid reaction. These findings are a common reactive response to bacterial infections and physiologic stress. Similarly, eosinophilia can be caused be parasitic infections or allergic reactions. Both may occur in response to certain medications. However, similar findings are seen in neoplastic disorders, such as chronic myelogenous leukemia (CML) or eosinophilic leukemia. When a "left shift" is accompanied by nucleated RBCs, the pattern is called a leukoerythroblastic reaction and may indicate a space-filling or myelophthisic lesion, such as fibrosis or metastatic carcinoma.

STANDARDS OF CARE

- A peripheral blood smear review should be performed for CBCs with leukocyte counts great than $50 \times 10^3/\mu L$ or with automated WBC differential results indicating the presence of greater than 2% immature granulocytes. Particular attention should be paid to the distribution of immature cells and the presence of increased atypical basophils and blasts.
- When analyzing CBC results, care should be taken to look for characteristics that are unusual for reactive neutrophilic leukocytosis before establishing this diagnosis. These may include anemia, thrombocytopenia or marked thrombocytosis, and basophilia, which could point to neoplastic disorders.
- There should be a low threshold for ordering a karyotype or fluorescence in situ hybridization (FISH) for *BCR/ABL1* on peripheral blood in a patient with neutrophilic leukocytosis. The presence of $t(9;22)$ by either of these techniques is diagnostic of CML.
- FISH testing for translocations involving PDGFRA and PDGFRB should be performed for any patient who meets the criteria of hypereosinophilic

syndrome, such as unexplained eosinophilia greater than 1,500/μL, especially if there is evidence of eosinophil-mediated organ damage.

ERRORS IN THE EVALUATION OF LYMPHOCYTIC LEUKOCYTOSIS

Failure to pay careful attention to clinical history and peripheral blood smear morphology, and selective use of ancillary tests, such as flow cytometry, when trying to distinguish between infectious/inflammatory conditions and malignant disorders. Lymphocytic leukocytosis is a normal reaction to a host of infectious (particularly viral or mycobacterial) and inflammatory conditions. Reactive lymphocytosis is often accompanied by a variety of changes in lymphocyte morphology. In addition, the number and morphology of lymphocytes vary with the patient's age. It is sometimes a challenge to distinguish these physiologic changes from those associated with chronic or acute lymphocytic leukemias.

STANDARDS OF CARE

- Absolute lymphocytosis should prompt manual review of the peripheral blood smear to help distinguish a reactive from a neoplastic process. Particular care should be taken in young children, in whom normal immature lymphocytes may circulate.
- The differential diagnosis of atypical lymphocytosis should always include reactive and infectious conditions, such as pertussis, ehrlichiosis, and infectious mononucleosis. These conditions should be ruled out by a careful clinical history, physical examination, and appropriate laboratory testing prior to a diagnosis of or referral for leukemia or lymphoma.
- In difficult cases, flow cytometry should be used to help distinguish reactive lymphocytosis from leukemia or lymphoma.

ERRORS IN THE DIAGNOSIS OF MYELODYSPLASIA

Failure to accurately distinguish true myelodysplastic syndrome (MDS) from its morphologic mimics. MDS is a clonal neoplasm of myeloid precursors characterized by peripheral cytopenias of myeloid, erythroid, and/or platelet lineages due to ineffective hematopoiesis. This leads to cytopenia-associated complications, including susceptibility to infection, anemia, and bleeding diathesis. Additionally, there is increased risk for the development of acute myeloid leukemia. Because peripheral blood and/or bone marrow elements generally exhibit morphologic dysplasia, diagnosis of MDS relies heavily on morphologic examination of peripheral blood and bone marrow aspirate smears. However, dysplasia is not a specific finding. It can be seen in a number of other disorders that exhibit clinical and laboratory findings similar to those of MDS, but for which the treatment and prognosis are much less severe.

STANDARDS OF CARE

▪ A complete nutritional study should be performed when investigating any new-onset macrocytic anemia. These studies should include tests for vitamin B_{12}, serum and RBC folate, copper, and zinc. RBC folate levels should be obtained before RBC transfusion.

▪ Bone marrow biopsy should be avoided if there is evidence of nutritional deficiency. If a bone marrow biopsy is performed, it is important to recognize that nutritional deficiencies can cause profound morphologic dysplasia. Thus, these findings should not be used as sole evidence of MDS. In fact, cytogenetic abnormalities may transiently be present due to B_{12} or folate deficiency as well.

▪ Morphologic dysplasia, such as Pelger–Huet cells, can be caused by a number of conditions other than MDS. Thus, one should rule out inherited, infectious, inflammatory, and nutritional causes before rendering a definitive diagnosis of MDS.

▦ MDS is almost always associated with one or more cytopenias. Caution should be exercised in the evaluation for MDS if the patient has a normal or near-normal CBC. In many cases, a repeat CBC after a period of time should be performed before proceeding with an invasive procedure such as a bone marrow biopsy.

HEMATOLOGY: PLATELETS

ERRORS IN THE EVALUATION OF THROMBOCYTOPENIA

Failure to recognize spurious causes of thrombocytopenia. The differential diagnosis of thrombocytopenia is broad and can involve defects in both bone marrow production of platelets and peripheral destruction or consumption of platelets. In either case, thrombocytopenia can indicate a significant bleeding risk and may be a marker of a serious underlying disorder. For these reasons, an accurate platelet count is crucial to clinical decision making. However, spuriously low platelet counts occur due to both technical and physiologic causes. It is important to recognize spurious causes of thrombocytopenia and rule them out by careful evaluation of a peripheral blood smear to prevent unnecessary procedures and incorrect diagnoses.

STANDARDS OF CARE

▦ Any new finding of thrombocytopenia should be evaluated by review of the peripheral blood smear. This will help rule out various artifacts, including platelet clumping and platelet satellitosis, which falsely reduce platelet counts produced by automated hematology analyzers. Review of the blood smear will also alert the physician to the presence of large platelets.

Platelet indices, including mean platelet volume (MPV) and the immature platelet fraction (IPF), should be used in conjunction with the platelet count to help determine whether thrombocytopenia is related to production defects or peripheral destruction. It can also help distinguish immune thrombocytopenia (ITP) from less common congenital disorders.

Patients with macrothrombocytopenia that shows uniformity in platelet size should be evaluated with a thorough personal and family history to evaluate for the possibility of a MYH9-related platelet disorder.

ERRORS IN THE EVALUATION OF THROMBOCYTOSIS

Failure to rule out all other causes of thrombocytosis prior to making a diagnosis of myeloproliferative disease. Thrombocytosis may be the first sign of a myeloproliferative disease, such as essential thrombocythemia or primary myelofibrosis, in an as yet asymptomatic patient. However, platelet counts can be elevated in many reactive conditions, including infection, trauma, surgery, and iron deficiency, among others. In addition, platelet counts can be incorrectly presumed to be elevated when a source of small interfering fragments approximately the size of a platelet are present in the blood.

STANDARDS OF CARE

A peripheral blood smear should be reviewed for all patients with a new diagnosis of thrombocytosis in order to confirm that the platelet count is likely to be correct, and to exclude possible spurious causes of a high platelet count.

▓ Thrombocytosis in the presence of iron deficiency should be considered reactive. Additional evaluation for thrombocytosis should not be performed unless the platelet count does not normalize with iron therapy.

▓ Other causes of reactive thrombocytosis should be excluded before referring a patient for evaluation of possible myeloproliferative disease.

▓ An "abnormal platelet distribution" flag from a hematology analyzer or a rapid, significant change in platelet count should trigger a manual peripheral blood smear review and platelet count estimate.

▓ In situations where tumor lysis is a possibility, leukocyte fragments should be excluded as a possible cause of an inaccurate platelet count before any procedures are performed to evaluate the patient for thrombocytosis.

IMMUNOLOGY: AUTOIMMUNE AND COMPLEMENT TESTING

ERRORS IN THE INTERPRETATION OF ANTINUCLEAR ANTIBODY TESTS

Failure to properly define the fluorescence pattern and titer of antinuclear antibody (ANA). ANAs are autoantibodies directed against antigens found in the nucleus of many different cell types. These antigens include double-stranded DNA (dsDNA), centromere proteins, histones, topoisomerases, and constituents of the small nuclear ribonucleoproteins (snRNPs), among others. ANAs are most often detected in patients with autoimmune collagen vascular diseases, including systemic lupus erythematosus (SLE), systemic sclerosis, Sjögren syndrome, inflammatory myopathies, and mixed connective tissue disease, although they can be seen to some degree in other disorders and occasional healthy patients. They are most commonly detected by indirect fluorescence assay (IFA) using standardized cultured human cells, such as Hep-2 cells. When positive, the fluorescence appears as distinct patterns in the interphase of mitotic cells, and these patterns correlate with specific nuclear antigens and specific collagen vascular diseases. The most common patterns are smooth/homogeneous, speckled, centromeric, and nucleolar, although some laboratories recognize additional patterns. Positive results are typically reported with the pattern and a titer, which is the highest dilution of serum at which fluorescence is detected. Properly recognizing and defining the fluorescence pattern and titer are paramount and allow for further evaluation for a patient with a specific autoimmune disease.

Positive ANAs are often followed by testing for extractable nuclear antigens (ENAs), which represent the specific antigens targeted by ANAs. Many ENAs have been described, but most laboratories test for common subsets that have particular disease associations, some of which are listed in Table 3.1. ENA testing is typically performed using an enzyme immunoassay (EIA) platform.

STANDARDS OF CARE

- ANA testing should be performed only in patients for whom there is a high clinical suspicion of collagen vascular disease based on defined diagnostic guidelines. It should not be used as a general screening test. This approach will increase positive predictive values and decrease false-positive results.
- Even when ordered appropriately, ANA results must be interpreted in the proper clinical context. Diagnosis of collagen vascular disease should not be based on ANA testing alone, but in concert with clinical findings and supportive radiographic and laboratory testing.
- Testing for specific ENAs should be restricted to patients known to have a positive ANA test.

Table 3.1: Extractable Nuclear Antigens

ENA Name	Antigen Target	ANA Pattern	Disease Association
Anti-dsDNA	Native DNA	Smooth/homogeneous	SLE
Antihistone	Histones	Smooth/homogeneous	SLE (especially drug-induced)
Anti-Sm	Ribonucleoprotein	Speckled or smooth	SLE
Anti-Ro (SS-A)	Ribonucleoprotein	Speckled	Sjögren syndrome or SLE
Anti-La (SS-B)	Ribonucleoprotein	Speckled	Sjögren syndrome or SLE
Anti-U1-RNP	Ribonucleoprotein	Speckled	Mixed connective tissue disease
Anti-Scl-70	DNA topoisomerase	Speckled or nucleolar	Systemic sclerosis
Anticentromere	Centromere proteins	Centromeric	Limited scleroderma

ERRORS IN THE INTERPRETATION OF THE RHEUMATOID FACTOR TEST

Failure to interpret rheumatoid factor (RF) results in clinical context or to rule out other associated diagnoses before making a diagnosis of rheumatoid arthritis (RA). RF is often elevated in the plasma or serum of patients with RA and has long been used as a tool in the diagnosis of this disease. However, the RF test is not specific. It can be elevated in a number of other conditions and occasionally in healthy patients.

STANDARDS OF CARE

- Serologic testing, whether using RF or anticyclic citrollinated peptide (anti-CCP), should be restricted to cases with intermediate diagnostic probability by history and physical examination.
- The RF test should not be relied on as the sole serologic test in the diagnosis of RA. Anticitrullinated peptide antibody (ACPA) tests, such as anti-CCP, which are more specific, should be utilized with or instead of RF.
- Positive RF tests should be interpreted carefully, as positive results are common in patients with other diseases, many of which have clinical features that significantly overlap with those of RA. Thus, these other disorders should be considered in the differential diagnosis until ruled out.

ERRORS IN THE INTERPRETATION OF ANTINEUTROPHIL CYTOPLASMIC ANTIBODY TESTS

Serologic tests to detect vasculitides can be positive in other, less severe nonvasculitic disorders and after exposure to certain drugs, and, thus, can be misdiagnosed as ANCA-associated vasculitides (AAVs). Antineutrophil cytoplasmic antibodies (ANCA) are autoantibodies most commonly associated with a group of severe systemic vasculitis syndromes, including Wegener's granulomatosis, Churg–Strauss syndrome, and microscopic polyangiitis, collectively known as ANCA-associated vasculitides (AAVs). The ANCA test is performed by an indirect immunofluorescence test in which patient serum is exposed to human neutrophils. In a positive test, application of a secondary fluorescently tagged antihuman IgG antibody reveals cytoplasmic positivity on formalin-fixed neutrophils. In ethanol-fixed neutrophils, one of two distinct patterns will emerge. Using this methodology, persistent cytoplasmic positivity is referred to as c-ANCA, while a perinuclear pattern is called p-ANCA. Autoantibodies against a number of different antigens can be responsible for ANCAs. However, the most common are myeloperoxidase (MPO) in p-ANCA and proteinase 3 (PR3) in c-ANCA, both of which are detected by EIA. Vasculitides are serious diseases with potentially high morbidity and mortality, and, thus, early definitive diagnosis is critical to effective therapy.

STANDARDS OF CARE

▓ ANCA tests should be ordered only in the proper clinical context; that is, when there is a high index of suspicion for AAV based on clinical and laboratory findings.

▓ Positive ANCA test results are nonspecific. Other causes of positive ANCA tests include medications, drugs, infections, and other nonvasculitic autoimmune diseases (eg, inflammatory bowel disease or autoimmune hepatitis). These must be ruled out before a diagnosis of AAV is rendered. This approach will decrease the probability of inappropriate diagnosis and therapy.

▓ Regardless of serologic results, a diagnosis of AAV should not be rendered in the absence of appropriate clinical, laboratory, and/or histologic evidence of disease. This is of particular concern when there is discordance between negative ANCA test results by immunofluorescence and positive anti-MPO or anti-PR3 results by EIA. Conversely, a positive ANCA test result is not required to make a presumptive diagnosis of AAV if the clinical suspicion is high.

ERRORS IN THE INTERPRETATION OF COMPLEMENT TESTING

Failure to differentiate between low complement levels from consumption and inherited deficiencies of complement proteins. The complement system is a series of blood proteins produced by the liver that act in concert with the innate and adaptive immune systems to clear pathogens. In a pathway in which proteins are sequentially activated in a cascade, complement proteins act variously to lyse cells, to opsonize organisms for phagocytosis, and to activate the immune system by acting as chemoattractants for leukocytes. In clinical practice, measurement of the complement system is used to diagnose deficiencies in the complement system. Low complement levels can be found in patients with congenital complement deficiencies and in those with increased formation of immune complexes. These include autoimmune disorders, such as SLE, and in renal diseases, especially various types of glomerulonephritis. In these cases, low complement levels are caused by consumption, as immune complexes activate the complement system. For this reason, complement measurement can also be used to monitor disease activity.

Common complement measurements include hemolytic complement activity, or CH50, which measures total complement pathway activity by assessing the ability of the patient serum to lyse sheep RBCs. Antigenic tests for total serum levels of complement factors C3 and C4 are also available.

STANDARDS OF CARE

▨ In cases with low C3 or C4 levels or a low CH50, non-immune complex causes of hypocomplementemia should be considered before making a definitive diagnosis of genetic complement deficiencies.

▨ When using complement activity and complement factor levels to monitor disease activity in immune complex–mediated disorders, trends in test result values are more significant than single values. This is especially true in patients who are pregnant or who have concomitant inflammatory disorders, for whom a significant decrease in complement levels can signal increased disease activity, even if the complement levels are still within the normal range.

IMMUNOLOGY: IMMUNOGLOBULINS

ERRORS IN THE EVALUATION OF PROTEIN ELECTROPHORESIS

Failure to define the heavy and light chain constituents of an "M Spike" that occurs during protein electrophoresis. Protein electrophoresis is a technique by which serum or urine proteins are separated by application of an electrical field to proteins loaded on a semisolid matrix. The resolution varies by assay, but proteins typically resolve into five distinct regions, representing albumin and alpha-1, alpha-2, beta, and gamma globulins. The concentration of each band is determined by densitometry. Because the shapes and relative concentrations of each band differ in a variety of pathologic conditions, protein electrophoresis can be a useful adjunctive diagnostic test for many diseases. However, its primary purpose is the detection, measurement, and monitoring of monoclonal immunoglobulin generated by plasma cell neoplasms. Monoclonal immunoglobulins appear as a sharp spike, typically in the gamma region on electrophoresis. This so-called "M spike" can be further analyzed by immunofixation electrophoresis, and this evaluation is required to define the heavy and light chain constituents of this abnormal band so that they can be followed in subsequently collected specimens.

STANDARDS OF CARE

▤ Blood collected for serum analysis must be allowed to adequately clot prior to centrifugation and electrophoresis. Failure to do so may lead to contamination by plasma proteins, such as fibrinogen, that can confound interpretation of the serum protein electrophoresis.

▤ Immunofixation electrophoresis should be performed for any positive or suspicious band on electrophoresis to determine if the band represents an immunoglobulin and to potentially characterize its identity for follow-up studies.

▤ Immunofixation, at least for light chains, should be performed on all follow-up studies to detect low levels of persistent monoclonal immunoglobulin.

▤ The presence of any abnormal bands should be carefully interpreted in the context of the patient history. A history of stem cell transplant, acute-phase reaction, hemolysis, or iron deficiency should be noted to aid in distinguishing bona fide M-spikes from oligoclonal bands and other confounding bands that can mimic M-spikes.

▤ In screening for myeloma, both serum and urine electrophoresis should be performed to aid in the detection of light chain–only myeloma.

ERRORS IN THE ANALYSIS OF FREE LIGHT CHAINS

Failure to exercise caution in the interpretation of light chain concentrations in the urine of patients with renal insufficiency. Despite equal stoichiometry of heavy and light chains in intact immunoglobulin, plasma cells produce more light chains than heavy chains. Consequently, free light chains circulate in the blood and are excreted into urine. Both kappa and lambda free light chains can be measured by nephelometry. Their absolute values and the ratio between kappa and lambda light chains can be used as surrogate markers for monoclonal immunoglobulin in the diagnosis and monitoring of plasma cell myeloma. However, because they are cleared by the kidney, caution must be exercised in the interpretation of light chain concentrations in the urine of patients with renal insufficiency.

STANDARDS OF CARE

▓ Serum free light chains must always be interpreted in the proper clinical context. In particular, elevated free light chains and high kappa:lambda ratios should be interpreted with caution in patients with renal insufficiency.

▓ Serum free light chains should not be evaluated independent of protein electrophoresis. While the light chain assays are a good screening tool, definitive diagnosis of monoclonal gammopathy requires the presence of an M-spike on serum and/or urine electrophoresis.

ERRORS IN THE ANALYSIS OF CRYOGLOBULINS

Failure to obtain reliable identification and quantification of a cryoglobulin because the sample was not stored at a constant temperature of 37°C prior to analysis. Cryoglobulins are serum immunoglobulins that precipitate at temperatures lower than normal body temperature. They are classified as three different types. Type I cryoglobulins are single monoclonal immunoglobulins, often associated with B cell or plasma cell neoplasms. Type II cryoglobulins are mixtures of polyclonal and monoclonal immunoglobulins. Type III cryoglobulins are polyclonal IgM. Mixed cryoglobulins (types II and III) are often associated with chronic viral infections, typically hepatitis C. Precipitation of cryoglobulins in serum can activate complement, leading to an inflammatory vasculitis. Cryoglobulins are measured by allowing them to precipitate at 4°C, quantifying the volume of cryoglobulin (cryocrit), and analyzing the cryoglobulin content by protein electrophoresis.

STANDARDS OF CARE

▫ Samples drawn for cryoglobulin assays must be placed promptly in a 37°C water bath for transport, and then handled and centrifuged at 37°C within the laboratory. Samples should not be allowed to cool below 37°C until after centrifugation to prevent loss of precipitated cryoglobulins from the specimen prior to analysis.

▫ Samples for cryoglobulin assays should not be drawn from a patient receiving intravenous heparin. Also, samples should be drawn from a peripheral vein, rather than from an intravenous line. If a sample must be drawn from an intravenous line, the first 10 mL of blood should be discarded prior to collection of the sample.

BIBLIOGRAPHY

Aletaha D, Neogi T, Silman AJ, et al. Rheumatoid arthritis classification criteria: an American College of Rheumatology / European League Against Rheumatism collaborative initiative. *Arthritis Rheum.* 2010;62:2569–2581.

Althaus K, Greinacher A. MYH-9-related platelet disorders: strategies for management and diagnosis. *Transfus Med Hemother.* 2010;37:260–267.

Bain BJ. *Haemoglobinopathy Diagnosis.* 2nd ed. Oxford, UK: Blackwell Publishing; 2006.

Beck CE, Hall M. Rheumatoid factor and anti-CCP autoantibodies in rheumatoid arthritis: a review. *Clin Lab Sci.* 2008;21:15–18.

Bosch X, Guilabert A, Font J. Antineutrophil cytoplasmic antibodies. *Lancet*. 2006;368:404–418.

Caldwell CW, Everett ED, McDonald G, Yesus YW, Roland WE. Lymphocytosis of gamma/delta T cells in human ehrlichiosis. *Am J Clin Pathol*. 1995;103:761–766.

Csernok E, Lamprecht P, Gross WL. Clinical and immunological features of drug-induced and infection-induced proteinase 3-antineutrophil cytoplasmic antibodies and myeloperoxidase-antineutrophil cytoplasmic antibodies and vasculitis. *Curr Opin Rheumatol*. 2010;22:43–48.

Gattens M, Morilla R, Bain BJ. Teaching cases from the Royal Marsden and St. Mary's Hospitals. Case 24: striking lymphocytosis in a 2-year old girl. *Leuk Lymphoma*. 2004;45:851–852.

Glassy EF, ed. *Color Atlas of Hematology: An Illustrated Field Guide Based on Proficiency Testing*. Northfield, IL: CAP Press; 1998.

Hamilton KS, Standaert SM, Kinney MC. Characteristic peripheral blood findings in human ehrlichiosis. *Mod Pathol*. 2004;17:512–517.

Hoyer JD, Kroft SH, eds. *Color Atlas of Hemoglobin Disorders: A Compendium Based on Proficiency Testing*. Northfield, IL: CAP Press; 2003.

Hudnall SD, Molina CP. Marked increase in L-selectin-negative T cells in neonatal pertussis. *Am J Clin Pathol*. 2000;114:35–40.

Kavanaugh A, Tomar R, Reveille J, Solomon DH, Homburger HA. Guidelines for clinical use of the antinuclear antibody test and tests for specific autoantibodies to nuclear antigens. *Arch Pathol Lab Med*. 2000;124:71–81.

Kjeldsberg CR, ed. *Practical Diagnosis of Hematologic Disorders, Benign Disorders*. 4th ed. Chicago, IL: ASCP Press; 2006.

Meroni PL, Schur PH. ANA screening: an old test with new recommendations. *Ann Rheum Dis*. 2010;69:1420–1422.

Motyckova G, Murali M. Laboratory testing for cryoglobulins. *Am J Hematol*. 2011;86:500–502.

O'Connell TX, Horita TJ, Kasravi B. Understanding and interpreting serum protein electrophoresis. *Am Fam Physician*. 2005;71:105–112.

Pamuk GE, Pamuk ON, Orum H, Demir M, Turgut B, Cakir N. Might platelet-leucocyte complexes be playing a role in major vascular involvement of Behcet's disease? A comparative study. *Blood Coagul Fibrinolysis.* 2010;21:113–117.

Satoh M, Vazques-Del Mercado M, Chan EK. Clinical interpretation of antinuclear antibody tests in systemic rheumatic diseases. *Mod Rheumatol.* 2009;19:219–228.

Savige J, Pollock W, Trevisin M. What do antineutrophil cytoplasmic antibodies (ANCA) tell us? *Best Pract Res Clin Rheumatol.* 2005;19:263–276.

Schoorl M, Schoorl M, Linssen J, et al. Efficacy of advanced discriminating algorithms for screening on iron-deficiency anemia and β-thalassemia trait. *Am J Clin Pathol.* 2012;138:300–304.

Shihabi ZK. Cryoglobulins: an important but neglected clinical test. *Ann Clin Lab Sci.* 2006;36:395–408.

Simon HU, Klion A. Therapeutic approaches to patients with hypereosinophilic syndromes. *Semin Hematol.* 2012;49:160–170.

Swerdlow SH, Campo E, Harris NL, et al, eds. *WHO Classification of Tumours of Haematopoietic and Lymphoid Tissues.* Lyon, France: IARC; 2008.

Tefferi A, Gotlib J, Pardanani A. Hypereosinophilic syndrome and clonal eosinophilia: point of care diagnostic algorithm and treatment update. *Mayo Clin Proc.* 2010;85:158–164.

Vavricka SR, Burri E, Beglinger C, Degen L, Manz M. Serum protein electrophoresis: an underused but very useful test. *Digestion.* 2009;79:203–210.

Wahed A, Risin S. Issues with immunology and serology testing. In: Dasgupta A, Sepulveda JL, eds. *Accurate Results in the Clinical Laboratory: A Guide to Error Detection and Correction.* Amsterdam, Netherlands: Elsevier; 2013:295–304.

Willis MS, Monaghan SA, Miller ML, et al. Zinc-induced copper deficiency: a report of three cases initially recognized on bone marrow examination. *Am J Clin Pathol.* 2005;123:125–131.

Zandecki M, Genevieve F, Gerard J, Godon A. Spurious counts and spurious results on haematology analyzers: a review. Part I: platelets. *Int J Lab Hematol.* 2007;29:4–20.

CHAPTER 4
Clinical Chemistry

JAMES H. NICHOLS
CAROL A. RAUCH

SPECIMEN RECEIVING AND PROCESSING

The specimen receiving and processing area of the laboratory is the entry point for specimens into the laboratory. As the initial contact point, processing staff may examine a specimen and detect common preanalytical errors before the specimen is analyzed. Mislabeling, wrong tube types, transportation delays, and other mistakes can affect patient results. By detecting and correcting problems before the specimen is placed on an analyzer, staff can prevent clinical mismanagement based on erroneous results. Receiving a quality specimen is the first step toward ensuring a quality result.

PREANALYTICAL ERRORS

Labeling Errors

Specimen mix-ups may occur and can lead to reporting erroneous results, and in turn to adverse events for the patient. A large clinical laboratory receives thousands of specimens each day. Specimens can look alike, because blood in a common collection tube does not look different from another sample of blood in the same type of tube. The specimen label is the only means of distinguishing among specimens. Clinicians may envision their patient as the only one being analyzed by the laboratory, but in today's highly automated clinical laboratory, specimens are lined up and analyzed solely based on the label/barcode on the side of the tube. Often, an operator must retrieve individual specimens if they are needed for reanalysis or additional testing. Searching for a specific specimen among racks of similar specimens can be labor intensive, so automated processes that archive and manage specimen storage and retrieval can improve the laboratory's efficiency. These additional processes are also based on information contained on the specimen label. Thus, clinicians must ensure that patients are properly identified and specimens are uniquely and appropriately labeled before sending them to the laboratory.

Labeling errors can encompass a variety of mistakes beyond unlabeled specimens. Samples can be mislabeled with another patient's name or contain incorrect information, such as name misspelling or wrong demographics such as age or sex. Partially labeled specimens contain two appropriate identifiers, but may be missing important information, such as specimen source or date/time of collection. Illegible labels that have been smudged or partially destroyed are also commonly encountered. Institutions should have a specimen labeling policy to determine how labeling errors will be handled. Some cases may present unique situations that require individual consideration, despite the existence of a labeling policy.

Specimen labeling errors may not be immediately apparent. Errors with one specimen may implicate that specimen in a labeling error and bring errors for multiple specimens into question. Thus, processing staff need to be diligent of the potential for mistakes and verify the integrity of specimen identification with each and every specimen arriving in the laboratory.

Collection in the Incorrect Tube Additive

Failure to follow the recommended collection and processing instructions can compromise the quality of test results. Specimen collection tubes are color coded to indicate different additives. Some additives prevent clotting and allow the analysis of plasma, while other additives inhibit glycolysis and metabolism. Color-coded tubes may also contain a gel barrier that facilitates sample processing. These different collection tubes have different intended purposes and are generally not interchangeable. Certain tests may require specific types of collection tubes, processing, or transport prior to analysis.

Errors in Specimen Transportation

Delays in transportation or exposure of specimens to extreme temperatures during transit to a laboratory can affect test results. Laboratories need to provide recommendations for limiting the exposure of specimens to extreme temperatures prior to processing and analysis. Couriers should monitor environmental conditions to ensure that specimens are maintained within specified conditions. The quality of test results can be affected by preanalytical conditions.

Specimen Processing Errors

The technique and manner of specimen processing can impact the quality of laboratory analysis. Failure to separate cells from the serum/plasma portion of blood allows for continued cellular metabolism that leads to decreased glucose values. Exposure of specimens to air, or transport of specimens with bubbles through a pneumatic tube, can alter blood gas values. Vigorous mixing of blood prior to analysis can generate foaming, which can affect pipette volumes and also induce hemolysis. Laboratories need to consider the possibility of preanalytical errors and take steps to minimize these errors.

STANDARDS OF CARE

- The clinical need for a test cannot overlook the issue of correct specimen identity.
- The integrity of the specimen from identification through collection, analysis, and reporting of results must be maintained.
- If a sample with a labeling error is analyzed, the test results should be associated with a comment to warn those interpreting the results of the potential for a specimen mix-up.
- Institutions must have a specimen labeling policy to determine how labeling errors will be managed.
- When the identity of a test result comes into question after analysis, the laboratory should never move the test from one patient's medical record to another patient's medical record.
- Specimens should be labeled in the presence of a patient immediately after collection to ensure that the specimen label matches the positive patient identification.
- The laboratory should be directly involved in phlebotomy education to ensure that staff understand test requirements and preanalytical variation that can occur during specimen collection.
- A laboratory should provide recommendations for limiting the exposure of specimens to extreme environmental conditions and to delays during transportation prior to processing and analysis.

CORE CHEMISTRY

The modern clinical chemistry laboratory is highly automated. Specimens are barcoded during collection, and usually arrive at the laboratory ready for analysis. In a high-volume laboratory, an integrated system of instrumentation and specimen tracks connect the analyzers, identify the tests required from the specimen barcode label, then centrifuge, aliquot, and perform the entire analysis without human intervention. This automation greatly reduces the possibility of previously common analytical errors such as mixing up aliquots, ordering incorrect tests within the laboratory, making dilution errors, and reporting results to the wrong patient. Even for low-volume laboratories, automation in the latest models of instrumentation detects interferences from hemolysis, bilirubin, and lipemia that can affect certain results on individual specimens. These analyzers flag results to be held by the instrument management system pending review by the technologist prior to release to the ordering physician. Automated control processes can detect other analytical issues (e.g., calibration errors, out-of-range controls, and failed delta checks and critical value limits) and warn the technologist of potential errors. Thus, automation of laboratory analyzers is an essential tool that enables the technologist to identify those specimens with unusual characteristics and specimens that need repeat testing or separate handling. This improves the overall quality of testing.

However, automated analyzers are not foolproof, and good-quality test results require quality specimens. Mislabeled and mishandled specimens, inappropriate collection and transport, miscommunication, and misunderstanding of protocols and procedures can generate erroneous results that are not detectable by automated chemistry instrumentation. Careful attention to specimen quality is required both within the laboratory as well as outside of the laboratory. Preanalytical errors in test ordering, specimen collection, transportation, and processing, as well as postanalytical errors in delivery and communication of test results, contribute to overall error rates that are related to laboratory testing. These errors remain a concern even for the most automated of laboratories.

PREANALYTICAL ERRORS

Specimen Collection Errors

The manner of specimen collection can impact the quality of test results. Collection of specimens through indwelling catheters presents a deviation from routine phlebotomy practice. Clinical staff are tempted to utilize intravenous lines, because lines provide direct access to the patient's circulation, minimize patient discomfort from additional needlesticks, and are easier for the staff since there is no need for additional equipment or localization of veins. However, collection of specimens through a line poses a risk of contaminating the specimen with whatever fluid and, possibly, drugs being administered through the line. In addition, use of indwelling catheters to collect specimens increases the risk of specimen hemolysis, the lysis of red blood cells within the sample, which can affect some test results.

Metabolites, proteins, drugs, and other molecules can be unstable in a patient sample. Glucose, for example, will continue to be metabolized by red blood cells and white blood cells in the sample during transport to the laboratory prior to analysis. This sample will have lower glucose results than the patient's actual levels at the time of collection. A specimen collected in the right collection tube with the right anticoagulant can stabilize the analyte for more accurate results. Fluoride and oxalate, for example, can inhibit glucose metabolizing enzymes and stabilize glucose in a specimen over longer periods of time compared to a specimen without the preservative. Different additives are identified by manufacturers with characteristic colors for stoppers on the specimen tubes. Red-topped tubes are plain tubes with no additive, while green-stoppered tubes indicate heparin, purple stoppers contain ethylenediaminetetraacetic acid (EDTA), and gray stoppers have the glycolytic inhibitors, fluoride and oxalate. Collection of multiple tubes during the same specimen collection can risk contamination of tubes with anticoagulant from previous tubes in the same collection.

Phlebotomy technique can affect the quality of the specimen and test results. Collection of a specimen at the wrong time or without required patient preparation can give misleading test results. Inappropriate phlebotomy technique can lead to hemolysis and the need to recollect a specimen, with a delay in results.

Specimen Labeling Errors

Errors in labeling can cause misdirection of the specimen within the laboratory, the wrong tests to be performed, inappropriate processing of the specimen, and reporting of results to the wrong patient. In a highly automated laboratory, labeling and barcodes direct the processing, analysis, and reporting of results for each specimen. The specimen label is as important as the quality of the specimen inside the tube. Incorrect labeling can lead to loss or difficulty retrieving the specimen from storage for reanalysis or review at a future time.

Reporting laboratory results to the wrong patient can create problems. Systems that protect the integrity of a patient specimen throughout the entire testing process ensure that the label on the specimen matches the result reported to the medical record. When specimen labeling or patient identity is in question, requesting recollection of the specimen and not reporting a result are better than reporting the result to the wrong patient. Laboratory results become part of the permanent legal medical record of the patient, so the ordering physician should be consulted any time there is a question over the proper labeling or identification of a specimen (or an aliquot of the original specimen) during the testing process.

ANALYTICAL ERRORS

Many types of mistakes can happen in the laboratory including errors in aliquoting, pipetting, dilution, calibration, and result entry, as well as those related to instrumentation. The analysis of liquid quality control samples is one means of detecting and preventing errors in the clinical laboratory. A control is a stabilized sample, analyzed like a patient sample, to determine if the test system is properly functioning. Results from control specimens that are within a target concentration range can verify the ability of the test system (reagent, analyzer, environment, and operator) to produce quality results with each batch of specimens. Clinical laboratory quality control principles were adopted from the manufacturing industry where products on a factory line are periodically tested to ensure that they meet specifications. As bottles of reagents sit on an analyzer, chemical activity in the reagents can drift and degrade over time. The analysis of controls verifies the stability of the test system and provides for reliability in the test results. However, when quality control specimens fail to achieve expected results, the laboratory must determine which component failed, correct the problem, and reanalyze the controls and patient specimens before releasing results. Patient results must only be released to clinicians when control results are acceptable.

Changing the specimen from serum to urine, or even from plasma to serum, requires a new evaluation of method performance since the test system may behave differently with different types of specimens. Analytical methods are calibrated to be used for specific specimen types. Conversion from plasma and serum can alter the specimen matrix. Also, results may differ due to the preservatives that are added when using plasma specimens. Laboratories verify method performance prior to offering a test in routine clinical practice by examining the assay precision, accuracy, linearity, and population reference ranges on a specific type of specimen. Laboratories must retain data from such studies. Whenever there is a question about assay performance, the original data can be used to document initial performance of the test system, assist in troubleshooting, and determine if there has been continued stability of instrument performance.

POSTANALYTICAL ERRORS

The attending physician may have to quickly act on a critical value without having seen or examined a patient. Unfortunately, for convenience, tests may be ordered by residents under an attending physician's name, and nurses may order tests for patients under a physician's name in a clinic setting. In these scenarios, the ordering physician of record may not have examined or even know the patient when he receives a call from the laboratory to accept and immediately act on a critical result. Critical or alert values are test results that represent a life-threatening situation, and require immediate and interruptive calls to a physician or clinical staff member that can take medical action.

STANDARDS OF CARE

■ Phlebotomy through catheters should be reserved for those patients with truly poor vascular access, those at risk of bleeding complications from traditional phlebotomy, and other highly special clinical circumstance. If used, this technique must only be performed at the request of a physician, with full knowledge of the risks and benefits of catheter-collected specimens, and the person obtaining such a specimen must be fully trained in these special techniques and fully knowledgeable about the line. The specimen source must be indicated with the test result, and patterns associated with dilution or other problems must have comments associated with results so that clinicians can assess whether results match the findings expected clinically.

- At least two unique identifiers (full name, birth date, medical record number, or other identifier) must be used to confirm patient identification, and verify the information on the specimen label/barcode during specimen collection.
- Any failure involving control specimens must be fully evaluated to determine the cause, rather than assume that the failure was due to chance.
- Tests on body fluid specimens require specific method validation to verify adequacy of technical performance on that type of specimen. Test results on body fluids must not be reported verbally or disclaimed with comments, when a method used has not been verified or the system performance is unknown.
- Laboratories are required to immediately contact physicians with critical test results. Physicians must take responsibility for tests they order (or allow to be ordered under their name), and ensure follow-up on the results of all ordered tests.

THERAPEUTIC DRUG MONITORING/TOXICOLOGY

Drug analysis involves the testing of samples for medications, toxins, and poisons. The discipline of toxicology spans many medical applications of a drug test result. The test may be intended for forensic purposes where the result may be entered as legal testimony in a court of law. Such cases include criminal intoxication, driving while impaired, child custody, cause of death, workplace drug testing, and sports/athletic doping. Forensic testing requires samples to be collected under a chain of custody where the specimen handling from collection, transportation, analysis, and result reporting can be strictly documented. Chain of custody is a paper trail providing assurance of specimen identity and integrity in order to confirm that the specimen belongs to a specific individual, has not been tampered with, and that the associated test result can be legally defensible in a court of law. Toxicology testing can also be conducted for clinical purposes, such as in the acute care of an emergency department (ED) patient, prenatal care, rehabilitation, and pain management. Test results can be quantitative (numeric) or qualitative (positive/negative), and drug analysis can be conducted using a variety of specimen types including urine, blood, hair, nails, meconium, and gastric and other body fluids. Some toxicology tests are used to screen patients for broad classes of drugs, while confirmatory testing can accurately identify a specific drug or metabolite. Given the number of drug tests and medical uses for the results, ordering the right test for a given situation can be confusing. Part of the laboratory's role is to define testing options clearly, so that ordering clinicians can understand what test is appropriate in order to answer the specific medical question regarding their patients.

PREANALYTICAL ERRORS

Test Ordering Errors

While the concept of panel testing is convenient, the question arises whether the patient really needs all of the tests in the panel performed or whether panel testing simply increases the cost of care. Laboratories frequently offer panels of drug tests. This facilitates ordering of drug testing for the clinician, since staff can order 10 or more tests on a patient's sample with a single test selection. Manufacturers of drug tests also offer point-of-care drug tests in multiple test panel configurations for screening of patient samples without requiring complicated laboratory instrumentation. Such formats include urine collection cups with a panel of drug tests embedded in the cup. In this assay, the patient collects a specimen, and staff twists the lid of the container, inverts the sample, and reads the results several minutes later.

Interfacing between laboratories and clinical information systems is complicated because there are so many different combinations of office system products for clinical information and laboratory information systems (LISs). There is increasing demand for electronic medical records (EMRs) in efforts to improve the efficiency of health care and to reduce errors. The U.S. government has offered incentives to physician offices for adoption of electronic record systems. As clinics adopt electronic records, laboratory ordering and reporting systems for these clinics are also increasingly becoming paperless. Electronic interfaces can communicate test orders between the clinic and a laboratory, and these interfaces can allow test results to flow automatically into the patient's record as soon as they are available on the analyzers. Government incentives for adopting electronic records and increased demand have given rise to hundreds of different vendors offering information systems to physician offices. In this environment, generic interfaces are often created for specific vendor combinations that can be modified for the individual clinic needs. Adoption of electronic interfaces between a clinical record and a clinical laboratory without implementing necessary customization (at additional cost) can lead to the availability of a wider test menu than was previously offered with paper requisitions in the physician office practice.

Ordering a test without considering the intended use of the result can create problems. For toxicology, results can be used for screening patients in the ED, managing prenatal care, or determining whether a patient is compliant with his or her pain management plan and rehabilitation program. In the ED, physicians are determining the cause of unconsciousness, anxiety, or altered mental status, while in the pain management or rehabilitation program, patients may actively be trying to deceive the physician in order to continue abusing drugs or obtain a refill for a narcotic prescription. Prenatal care plans to promote healthy fetal development pose possible legal consequences with risk of newborn withdrawal and possible child social services involvement with drug abuse. Thus, there are different requirements for testing, and drug tests are methodologically not all equivalent. Acute clinical management requires fast results when there may not be time for confirmatory testing, if it takes place hours to days later. On the other hand, clinical care with rehabilitation, pain management, or tests with potential legal consequences necessitate confirmation prior to reporting and medical action.

Specimen Collection Errors

Drug test results can have significant impact on patients' lives. Positive test results for opiates, cocaine, tetrahydrocannabinol (THC), amphetamines, and phencyclidine each could indicate that a patient is abusing street drugs. Patients with positive drug tests may be noncompliant with treatment program contracts and could have their opiate prescriptions stopped. Positive test results on patients returning from leave (for work or home visitation) from a supervised rehabilitation home could be evidence of continued drug use. Test results may lead to dismissal from a live-in treatment program and possible reversal of probation for patients under court-ordered rehabilitation. Positive results for employment testing or after on-the-job accidents could lead to refusal to hire, job suspension, firing, or liability lawsuits.

In addition to all these potential consequences of a positive test, it must be understood that patients can adulterate or add substances to their urine sample after collection in an attempt to generate false-negative test results. Adulterants are not the only means that patients may use to thwart drug tests. Some patients may resort to substitution, the use of a synthetic urine, or submission of another patient's urine as their own sample.

In emergency management situations, failure to test the patient for drugs can lead to problems. Patients can present with altered mental status due to an organic disease process, such as low blood sugar or mental illness, from trauma, or, not uncommonly, a medication reaction. The physician must sort out what may be causing the symptoms and decide on a treatment plan. When drugs are involved, the laboratory must determine which drug among the thousands of possibilities the patient may have taken. Not only is the choice of specimen a consideration, notably urine versus blood, but also whether the analytical methods are sufficiently sensitive to detect the drug in question. Clues from the physical exam, past medical history, and the presence of pills or powders on the patient can narrow the list of potential medications for drug testing and help determine the appropriate analyses required for identification of an unknown substance.

ANALYTICAL ERRORS

The number of significant figures in a test result can lead to errors of interpretation. Too much detail by reporting of results to the tenths or hundredths decimal place can give the clinician overconfidence in the precision of the method. Too little detail and rounding of results may give the impression that the laboratory's analytical performance is worse than comparative methods. The laboratory director must find a balance to represent the precision of the method and minimize the risk of physician misinterpretation of test results.

POSTANALYTICAL ERRORS

While physicians may request preliminary screening test results to allow for immediate clinical decisions, this can lead to incorrect interpretation of results and inappropriate patient management. Screening tests are utilized to rapidly identify potentially positive samples, amid a large number of negative specimens, for additional confirmation testing. Screening tests are generally automated assays that require little technologist involvement, compared to confirmation testing such as mass spectrometry, which is more labor intensive and costly. Screening tests gain efficiency for the laboratory by confirming only positive samples, rather than performing a confirmation level test on every specimen arriving with a request for drug testing. Screening tests have limitations and can demonstrate false-positive results from common over-the-counter and prescribed medications. Confirmation of screen-positive specimens is especially required whenever test results may lead to legal or medical action. Unfortunately, confirmation testing is not available in every hospital laboratory, so the turnaround time for a test result may be several days. For critical and emergent patient management, test results are needed much sooner.

The cutoff concentration in a confirmatory test must closely match the screening test cutoff concentration. Otherwise patients that are positive by screening may be negative by confirmation. Drug screen results are generally reported qualitatively and have defined cutoff concentrations that allow discrimination of positive samples with concentrations at or above the cutoff level from negative samples with concentrations below the cutoff. Samples that screen positive can then be analyzed by a more specific method, like mass spectrometry, that can confirm the presence of individual drugs or metabolites.

Contacting an appropriate person who is willing to accept a critical drug test result can be challenging. Critical values are life-threatening results that require immediate, interruptive contact of the ordering physician, or their designee who can take clinical action. Laboratories are required by the Clinical Laboratory Improvement Amendments (CLIA) to contact a live person and document that communication of the critical result took place with read-back (to ascertain the accurate comprehension of the verbal result). Critical value communication is generally documented with the test result in the LIS or EMR.

Holding antibiotic doses until stat requests for vancomycin levels can be obtained is not usually necessary.

The controversy over whether vancomycin is linked to nephrotoxicity and ototoxicity alone, or in combination with other aminoglycoside antibiotics, has led to requests for stat testing from the laboratory. Clinicians often cannot obtain the vancomycin level results fast enough, and doses are being held for fear that the patient may be above the therapeutic range. Nurses are anxious to give the next dose, and want the drug level to confirm that the patient is not at an elevated level before giving the dose. However, in most cases, stat requests for vancomycin levels are unnecessary and the antibiotic doses do not need to be held.

STANDARDS OF CARE

- Physicians must be selective in ordering laboratory tests. Order what is medically necessary for a patient based on the symptoms and diagnosis. It is not appropriate to screen for an abnormality using large panels of tests. Manufacturers should provide the ability to select individual tests on their instrumentation instead of forcing panel configurations that encourage unnecessary tests.
- While grouping tests can facilitate physician ordering, panels of tests encourage overutilization of unnecessary testing.
- Laboratories must match test cutoffs for screening and confirmation tests for drug testing.
- Physicians and laboratories must consider the possibility of deception in drug testing. Patients can dilute, adulterate, or substitute their samples in order to generate false-negative drug test results.
- Laboratories must educate physicians on the limitations of drug screening tests, common sources of false-positive and false-negative test results.
- Results should only be reported to an appropriate number of significant figures. Assay performance should reflect technical and biologic variation and a laboratory must work with physicians to ensure

that reporting format matches the true assay performance and medical needs.

▦ Critical values are life-threatening results that require immediate, interruptive contact of the ordering physician or a designee who can take clinical action. Ordering clinicians must be aware of this expectation and accept responsibility for patient management.

▦ Clinicians should rarely treat solely based on the screening test results for drugs of abuse. Drug screens can have false-positive cross-reactivities that require confirmatory testing by a more specific method to appropriately identify a specific drug and metabolite.

▦ Administration of the next dose of antibiotics, especially vancomycin, should rarely be held pending laboratory results, creating a false need for laboratory urgency when, for most patients, a dose does not need to be held. Pharmacists should assist the laboratory in educating clinical staff on the proper timing of specimen collection and dose administration for therapeutic monitoring.

▦ Laboratories must understand their automated processes, work to maximize efficiency, and limit stat requests to those patients who urgently require the faster turnaround time.

POINT-OF-CARE TESTING

Point-of-care testing (POCT) refers to diagnostic laboratory testing conducted close to the site of patient care, outside of a central, or core, laboratory setting. POCT is generally conducted by clinical staff, such as physicians, nurses, emergency medical technicians, and respiratory therapists, without formal laboratory experience or background in laboratory testing. The advantage of POCT is the speed at which test results can be produced, because a specimen does not need to be transported to a laboratory for analysis and have results communicated from the laboratory back to the clinician for medical action. POCT is conducted in a variety of settings including operating rooms, intensive care units, physician offices, ambulances, and helicopters. POCT has even been conducted on the space shuttle. An increasingly diverse menu of rapid POCT is being marketed for testing, including blood gases, electrolytes, glucose, numerous infectious diseases, drugs of abuse, and hormones to assess fertility. These devices use a variety of testing methodologies: biosensors, immunochromatography, and now even molecular diagnostics. POCT has historically been perceived to be less reliable than core laboratory testing because of extra challenges posed in ensuring operator competence, quality control performance, appropriate analysis, and test result documentation. POCT is often viewed by clinical staff as a distraction from patient care and a laboratory task added onto an already overburdened nursing workload amid managing patients and staffing shortages on the clinical unit. Yet, POCT is not a threat to central laboratory analysis; it is an integral part of patient care and an extension of the laboratory when a centralized laboratory cannot deliver a fast enough turnaround time for results. The laboratory should facilitate understanding of medical need, how the test result will be utilized, and the various options available for laboratory testing to meet clinical needs. The laboratory is a resource for best practices and quality standards, and can assist nursing and clinical staff in achieving reliable results, no matter who performs the test and where the test is conducted. Optimal implementation, planning, procedures, and training strategies that incorporate POCT into patient management pathways assist physicians in ordering the appropriate test for the patient while delivering reliable results that meet regulatory requirements.

▓▓▓▓ **IMPLEMENTATION MISTAKES**

Failure to Recognize POCT Differences and Limitations

POCT is not always the best testing method in a hospital setting. The inability to obtain a fast turnaround of test results from a central laboratory is often the motivation to implement POCT on the nursing unit. The laboratory is seen as the limiting step to discharging patients from an ED or moving patients through the hospital. However, all laboratory methodologies have limitations and unique interferences that can generate misleading test results when utilized on the wrong patient populations or on incorrect specimen types. These limitations need to be considered when choosing POCT over central laboratory methodologies.

Using POCT to Solve Overly Complex System Problems

POCT, with its associated burden of operator training and competency, maintenance, reagent storage, and documentation considerations, can add unnecessary stress to a clinical setting. Why the test is needed and how the test result will be utilized in patient care decisions should be clearly defined before a faster result can be safely concluded to facilitate patient care. Measures of patient outcome should be benchmarked before and after implementation of POCT in order to determine if POCT improved patient outcome or simply complicated an already overly complex pathway of care. Sometimes streamlining the pathway of care is a better alternative than adding POCT.

Misunderstanding Regulatory Requirements

Failure to comply with testing regulations and certification can cause problems. The U.S. CLIAs of 1988 law mandates licensure of laboratories testing human patient samples where the test results will be utilized to make clinical decisions. Even laboratories performing simple POCT such as pregnancy, urine dipstick, or glucose meter tests must apply for a CLIA certificate, pay a fee every two years, follow manufacturer's instructions, and agree to be inspected. More complex testing than POCT requires additional documentation of operator training and competency, quality control, maintenance, and written policies for patient preparation, sample collection, processing, analysis, and result reporting.

Failure to understand where and how CLIA regulations apply. CLIA regulations apply to clinical laboratory testing. CLIA applies to tests conducted within a formal laboratory or outside of a laboratory, in a satellite or point-of-care setting. CLIA also applies to clinical samples from U.S. citizens that are analyzed within or outside of the United States. The analysis of forensic specimens, nonhuman specimens, such as veterinary samples, and research testing are exempt from the CLIA law. However, tests that lead to a change in patient management or medical decision making are considered to be regulated under CLIA even if those tests are conducted as part of a research study.

Failure to train staff to be competent and capable of obtaining performance that meets expected manufacturer specifications as approved by the FDA can cause problems. Although method verification is only required for nonwaived tests under the CLIA regulations, method verification is a good laboratory practice for all POCT regardless of the test complexity classification status. The site performing testing should know the method precision, bias, and reportable range of results, and verify the reference interval for normal results.

TEST ORDERING MISTAKES

Distinguishing POCT from Central Laboratory Tests

Uniformity in testing methodology between laboratories and POCT protocols is not always guaranteed, which can create confusion. As a general rule, POCT uses different methodology than instrumentation found in the central laboratory. Some tests may generate comparable test results, but other tests may give quite different results. Clinicians ordering a test need to understand the differences between available test methods, and the test names need to be clear enough to ensure that the physician is ordering the right test for his or her patient. Simply naming the test "stat" or "POCT" does not ensure that the physician understands the appropriate specific test limitations or that the results will actually meet an intended medical use of the test. Laboratories need to work with their information technology and sales/marketing departments to review how tests are displayed on electronic and written requisitions, and to ensure that test-specific information is readily available to the ordering clinician, especially if multiple options exist.

Overutilization of POCT

POCT can facilitate patient outcomes, but only if staff are available to act on the test results. If the ordering physician is away from the unit, and the POCT results sit in a patient's chart waiting for review, the intended benefit of a faster result is lost. Overutilization of POCT is a risk, because POCT is convenient to use on the nursing unit. It is easier than printing specimen labels and sending samples off to a central laboratory. Overutilization of POCT can be costly to hospitals because single-use tests are more expensive on a per-test basis than bulk reagents used in core laboratory testing. Without the benefits of improved patient outcome, performing POCT can waste both financial and staff resources in time spent performing the test outside the laboratory and documenting regulatory compliance. The decision to perform a test at the point-of-care or to send a sample to a central laboratory should be based on how the test result will be utilized in the care of the patient. POCT has a place in emergent management decisions for rapidly changing conditions, but orders for future POCT where the result is not linked to immediate care decisions should be carefully reviewed.

PREANALYTICAL ERRORS

Collecting Samples Through Indwelling Catheters

A majority of laboratory errors actually occur outside of the physical walls of the laboratory and involve preanalytical errors, such as errors in specimen collection, as well as postanalytical errors, such as delays in acting upon results and result misinterpretation. Quality test results require quality specimen collection. A POCT device cannot compensate for a poor-quality specimen. Indwelling catheters are a common source of specimen collection errors because they frequently involve fluid or drug contamination of the specimen.

Use of POCT on Alternative Samples

Problems can occur when changing the specimen type or intended use of the test. Staff may not realize that changing the specimen type or the intended use of the test (e.g., from monitoring for a disease to screening for a diagnosis) can change the CLIA complexity of a test and the number of additional activities that must be performed and documented for regulatory compliance. As an example, off-label use of POCT can raise the CLIA complexity of a test to a high-complexity level. High-complexity tests involve those developed by the laboratory or tests where the manufacturer's instructions have been modified. High-complexity tests require additional method verification and performance documentation.

Quality Control Mistakes

Failure to implement quality control procedures periodically can create problems. Quality control is the analysis of a liquid-stabilized sample, in the same manner as a patient sample, to determine if the performance of the test system, reagents, operator, and device meet quality specifications. Quality control is analyzed periodically to ensure the reliability of patient test results. Newer POCT devices have computerized data management that facilitates the collection of operator identification, patient, and test information at the time of analysis, and links that information to the test result. Data management systems that can automate the documentation of test and quality control results greatly assist in compliance with laboratory quality regulations, as staff can forget to analyze quality control and continue to test patients.

Sharing Operator Identification Numbers

POCT devices look simple, but there is no foolproof device. Like any laboratory test, errors can occur when devices are used incorrectly or testing is performed by untrained operators. Good laboratory practice requires the operator to read and follow the manufacturer's instructions. Inappropriate sample collection, poor timing, or result misinterpretation can lead to incorrect results. More complex devices requiring multiple steps for collection and analysis of specimens necessitate more detailed training and practice. CLIA regulations for professional use of a POCT device require documentation of initial operator training and, at minimum, annual checks of ongoing competency for CLIA moderate- and high-complexity tests. Keeping manual records for hundreds of operators can be time consuming and very challenging to maintain. Fortunately, newer POCT devices with computerized data management have the capability to lock out operators. This feature ensures that only trained and competent operators are providing testing. An operator must enter his or her own personal identification number before the device will unlock and allow patient testing.

ANALYTICAL ERRORS

Data Entry Errors With Patient Identification

Despite its advantages, data management creates the possibility for a new class of laboratory errors involving data entry mistakes. Data management provides a means of automating the data collection and documentation that ensure regulatory compliance. Each test result is linked to the date/time, serial number of the device, the operator, reagent lots, and quality control for the reagent and analyzer. With data management, there is a record of every test performed, successful or not, and error codes and action comments are captured when a test fails. Manual records inevitably miss the recording of some test results, and errors/repeated tests may not get documented.

Other Data Entry Errors

Data entry errors can occur with any step of the analytical process. Incorrect operator identification entry is detected by the device as an invalid or untrained operator attempting access and, if the feature is available, lock-out prevents patient testing. Patient identification errors, however, allow testing to occur, but the results become stuck in the POCT data management system. An invalid patient identifier tied to a test result that does not match an active patient medical record forces the data management system to search the admissions systems for that patient. If there is no match, the test result cannot be posted to the patient's record. Data entry errors can also occur in identification of control samples and reagent lots used for testing. These errors pose challenges to accurate compliance documentation.

Blind Operators

Failure to document that staff can perform the test and achieve a result that is within expected tolerance can cause problems. Training is more than simply orienting staff to the procedure. Staff must demonstrate that they can perform all ancillary tasks required to generate an accurate test result. Temperature monitoring, instrument maintenance, quality control testing, and result reporting/follow-up are all components of performing the test. Adequate performance of all steps of the testing process is necessary to demonstrate competency. This requires (1) direct observation of routine test performance; (2) monitoring the recording and reporting of results (including critical value communication); (3) review of intermediate test results and worksheets including quality control, proficiency testing, and maintenance records; (4) observation of instrument preventive maintenance and function checks; (5) assessment of test performance using previously tested specimens, internal correlation samples, and external proficiency testing samples; and (6) evaluation of trouble-shooting skills. All six of these criteria are now being reviewed by CLIA, The Joint Commission, and the College of American Pathologists (CAP) inspectors, as required elements of staff competency for CLIA nonwaived tests.

Temperature Monitoring and Reagent Storage Errors

Quality results require quality reagents. Test strips, kits, and control materials that are exposed to heat, cold, humidity, and other environmental extremes can degrade before being used in patient testing. Shipments of test kits can be exposed to heat during the summer and cold during the winter while sitting outdoors being loaded onto trucks and airlines for transit. Testing staff have no idea of the condition of the reagents upon receipt of a shipment. Thus, good laboratory practice dictates verifying the performance of kits within each shipment using previously analyzed specimens or specimens of known analyte concentration, such as control or proficiency testing samples. Once received, the responsibility for meeting manufacturer-recommended storage conditions falls on the laboratory and staff within the hospital where the reagents will be stored. For POCT reagents, some storage will occur on the nursing unit. Refrigerated reagents and controls must be stored according to manufacturer specifications, and corrective action must be taken when kit storage does not meet those specifications.

Failure to Follow Manufacturer's Directions

The large volume of tests performed and the need to conduct the analysis the same way, from step A to step B to step C without variance, each time, poses a risk for error. POCT is challenged by the large number of staff involved in the process. In an average institution, there may be dozens of locations utilizing hundreds of devices with thousands of operators. With the pressures of clinical care and patient management, human nature will strive to gain efficiencies by using shortcuts to work around strict procedures and find ways to reduce the time staff spends on the test while maximizing time with the patient. No one intends for bad results to happen. Clinical staff rarely understand the consequences of varying the procedures for point-of-care tests, or the effect that shortcuts may have on test results.

Taking Procedural Shortcuts

Procedural shortcuts can lead to errors. Shortcuts may occur within one test procedure, or they may occur across several tests; the latter type is more insidious to identify the cause and troubleshoot. Because POCT devices offer limited menus, several tests and devices are often employed at the same time on a nursing unit to meet medical needs. Having a single sample shared for performing multiple POCTs may create unpredictable types of errors.

Sample Application Mistakes

Sample volume can affect a test result. Application of too much sample on a POCT pregnancy test strip, for instance, may flood the kit, dilute the antibody conjugate, and create problems with ability to detect and interpret the result. Too little sample may lead to failure of adequate specimen flow and not allow test and control reagents to react with their respective zones on the test. Staff may know and attempt to follow the proper procedure but take liberties with sample application, often because of a limited amount of sample or the medical urgency for the test.

POSTANALYTICAL ERRORS

Infrequent Operators

Individuals who perform POCT tests infrequently are more likely to perform the test incorrectly. Mistakes can occur with test interpretation, especially for manual, visually interpreted POCT. Staff should verify the method of interpretation and appropriate timing of test development. Lighting can affect color changes. Fluorescent, incandescent, and even natural sunlight can alter shades of color in the operator's visual interpretation of results. Storage of kits near a window can degrade colored conjugates within the kits, so tests should be protected from bright light by storing kits within the manufacturer's protective packaging until just before use. Over- and under-incubating of the sample can lead to false-positive and false-negative test interpretations.

Distinguishing POCT From Central Laboratory Results

POCT is a different method from core laboratory testing, and the results will differ as well, even when the exact same sample is used for both tests. Each methodology has unique interferences and limitations. A POCT glucose result is not the same as a result from another glucose method, and POCT sodium may not be the same result as that obtained by other sodium methods. Misinterpretation can occur if results from different methodologies are intermixed.

Reassessing Need for POCT

The laboratory's failure to regularly interact with the physicians utilizing POCT can cause problems. As a rapid diagnostic test, POCT should be meeting an urgent medical need for results on the unit that cannot be met by central laboratory turnaround times. Even routine POCT should periodically be reassessed for clinical need to ensure that the POCT test is truly required, particularly in light of ongoing improvements in central laboratory diagnostics.

STANDARDS OF CARE

■ The laboratory must collaborate with medical staff to determine the need for POCT laboratory tests, turnaround times, and how the test result will drive further patient care decisions. The availability of pneumatic tubes for specimen transport, the proximity of the unit to the laboratory, and the specific instrumentation available in the laboratory all differ from one hospital to another. Whether to offer a test at the point-of-care is thus a unique decision for each facility, based on the overall needs and ability of the laboratory to meet those needs with traditional laboratory instrumentation.

■ While the goal of POCT may be a common, shared reference range, differences between POCT and central laboratory results exist and must be considered when making medical decisions. Test orders and results for POCT and the central laboratory as well as other methods for the same test (e.g., blood gas analyzers) should be separate and distinguishable in the patient's medical record.

■ Cost issues must not be the only consideration when POCT is requested. If a faster turnaround for POCT results leads to quicker discharge decisions, facilitates movement of patients through the health system, frees operating and procedure rooms, and opens beds for waiting patients, the additional cost of POCT may translate to better overall patient outcomes.

■ The laboratory should be involved with POCT as a resource for promoting good laboratory practices, quality control, documentation, and regulatory compliance.

■ Manual tests are more prone to errors. Data management should be utilized to improve regulatory compliance and to automate the documentation and transfer of POCT results to the patient's medical record.

■ Written procedures, regular performance of quality control, and operator training/competency are all required components of good laboratory practice for POCT.

■ Medical need should drive the implementation of POCT, and POCT should be included as a component of quality patient care where indicated.

ENDOCRINE/TUMOR MARKERS/SPECIAL CHEMISTRY

Endocrine testing concerns the analysis of hormones, peptides, and other compounds secreted by the glands of the body. Hormones can be proteins, such as thyroid-stimulating hormone (TSH) and parathyroid hormone, or smaller molecules such as thyroxine or cortisol. Endocrine tests sometimes measure a hormone directly, but in other instances may analyze compounds affected by hormones. For example, in diabetes mellitus, primarily a disease of insulin deficiency or insufficient insulin action at tissue receptors, clinicians diagnose and manage the disorder through analysis of glucose levels rather than through direct measurement of circulating insulin levels. Endocrine tests are utilized to diagnose and manage disorders of the pituitary, thyroid, parathyroid, adrenals, ovaries, testes, and other organs of the body. Due to the variety of different compounds related to endocrine function, testing for endocrine disorders involves a variety of methodologies. Competitive immunoassays that rely on the binding of hormones and metabolites to specific antibodies in the test reagent are often utilized. Glucose is measured by enzyme-specific reagents with colorimetric endpoints. Immunoassays and spectrophotometric assays can be automated on laboratory instrumentation, but more manual methods, such as radioimmunoassay and enzyme-linked immunosorbent assays, are also employed for analysis of hormones and compounds. Failure to follow basic laboratory practices with specimen labeling, collection, transportation, analysis, and result reporting can lead to test result errors. In addition, some hormones and compounds are unstable in patient samples, so appropriate specimen collection and handling are of particular concern to ensure accurate detection and quantitation of the amount of hormone in the patient's sample.

PREANALYTICAL ERRORS

Failure to correctly identify a patient using multiple identifiers is substandard. Proper patient identification is paramount to good laboratory practice. The assurance of specimen-labeling integrity starts with the proper identification of the patient. Current standards of practice dictate the use of two unique identifiers as part of the patient identification process. These may include full name, birth date, medical record number, social security number, or other form of individual identification. As the first step in the testing process, the phlebotomist should check that the patient's name matches his or her identification, particularly when physician orders, test results, and insurance or other billing are tied to patient identification.

The matrix of a specimen is affected by the type of anticoagulant used for specimen collection, and plasma is different from serum. Specimens can be collected in blue-stoppered tubes (citrate for coagulation), purple-stoppered tubes (EDTA for cell counts), green-stoppered tubes (heparin for blood gases and chemistries), or gray-stoppered tubes (fluoride and oxalate for glucose analysis). All of these tubes will generate a plasma sample when centrifuged to separate the cells. However, not all of the anticoagulants are equivalent and will have variable effects on certain tests. Laboratories need to ensure that the specimen collection tube and specific anticoagulant have been validated for the particular test ordered.

Measuring insulin levels instead of analyzing blood glucose levels in testing for diabetes is not good practice. Diabetes mellitus is a disease of increasing concern in developed countries due to the prevalence of obesity and lack of exercise. Diabetes is a disorder of insulin deficiency or decreased insulin action at the tissues, characterized by high blood glucose levels. Although diabetes is considered an endocrine disorder, diabetes is diagnosed and managed through the analysis of glucose levels rather than direct measurement of insulin concentration.

Overutilization of thyroid-related tests can lead to mistakes in result interpretation and can contribute to increased costs of health care. The ordering of thyroid tests can be confusing. Laboratories can offer TSH, thyroxine (T4), triiodothyronine (T3), free thyroxine (fT4), free triiodothyronine (fT3), T3 resin uptake (T3RU), free thyroxine index (FTI), thyroglobulin (Tg), thyroglobulin antibodies (TgAb), thyroxine-binding globulin (TBG), and thyroid peroxidase antibodies (TPOAb) in their thyroid function test menu. Clinicians must be familiar with each of these tests and their limitations to pick the right test to address their diagnostic questions. The desire to order more thyroid-related tests than needed is tempting, given the large number of available thyroid-related tests.

ANALYTICAL ERRORS

Drug interferences and other problems can affect analysis. Immunoassays incorporate specific antibodies to detect an analyte in a patient's specimen. There can be a number of interferences, including drugs and cross-reactive compounds, that can affect test results. False-positive elevations in test results can occur from these interferences and cause incorrect test result interpretations and patient mismanagement.

POSTANALYTICAL ERRORS

The manner in which a test result is displayed can impact test interpretation. Clear display of test results is especially important when a series of specimens is collected at the same time or in close succession as part of a patient procedure.

STANDARDS OF CARE

- At least two unique identifiers must be used to confirm patient identification and verify the information on the specimen label/barcode during specimen collection.
- Laboratories must arrange for appropriate specimen collection, prompt processing, and analysis of samples to ensure appropriate recovery of physiologic levels of unstable analytes in a patient's sample.
- Overutilization of laboratory tests can lead to incidental abnormal results that can be misleading and lead to unnecessary follow-up with increased cost of health care.
- Laboratories should be aware of the possibility of false-positive test results due to heterophilic antibodies and recommend that physicians always interpret test results in conjunction with the patient's symptoms and clinical condition.

■ Diagrams and visual tools assist the interpretation of test results, especially when multiple specimens are collected sequentially during a patient procedure.

LABORATORY INFORMATION SYSTEMS/ INFORMATICS

The LIS is more than a database that stores all of the test results generated by the laboratory. An LIS acts as an intermediary to the clinical information systems and EMRs utilized by clinical staff to manage patient care. Most physicians do not have direct access to the LIS and never work within that system. In the clinical laboratory, results must be collected from the analyzing instruments by the LIS, managed, and transmitted for display to the physicians in the EMR. The interfaces between the laboratory analyzer and LIS to the final EMR can each be sources of error that laboratories need to consider. As data are electronically transmitted from the laboratory to the hospital and onward to other electronic databases and records in the physician's office, insurance companies, government agencies, and even personal health records, test names can be confused, decimal points moved, and comments misinterpreted. A new responsibility of the laboratory in the age of paperless records is verifying that the result is correctly displayed for the ordering physician and that it can be appropriately interpreted after it is transferred through the variety of electronic systems.

PREANALYTICAL ERRORS

Ordering Mistakes

Misleading test names can cause the wrong test to be ordered and lead to specimen recollection, repeat testing, result corrections, and duplicate ordering on an individual or, worse, systematically throughout a health care system. Test names typically convey both the purpose and utility of the laboratory analysis. Test names can also be confusing, especially when there are several closely related tests that differ in method limitations, sensitivity, or clinical application. The laboratory has a responsibility to clarify for both ordering physicians and information system programmers which test result is the correct one being reported.

Test names can also be confusing in the order and result interfaces between electronic record systems. A physician may want a specific test and use one name on the requisition, but the reference laboratory performing the test may call the test by a different name or offer several tests with similar names. Mapping test requests in one system to specific tests on a menu in another system is part of the programmer's job when developing communication interfaces between different electronic systems. The processing staff in the specimen-receiving area of the laboratory must further determine the appropriate test to select when translating test requests and written requisitions as they arrive in the laboratory. Placing test requests over an LIS interface or selection of the wrong test because the correct name is not known to the ordering provider can both be sources of error.

When the LIS operator ignores a warning or the system allows the operator to bypass built-in safety checks, errors can occur. Electronic databases are created to facilitate both data entry and retrieval. An LIS can provide internal checks to warn of potential errors and caution the operator to verify the data before continuing.

ANALYTICAL ERRORS

In many ways, laboratory instrumentation has become so automated that technologists can sometimes forget what they need to do manually because the analyzer has been performing it automatically for a long time. With electronic information systems, many tasks routinely conducted by technologists are now automated. Lipemia, icterus, and hemolysis, common interfering substances, are now detected by the instrument automatically. Specimen clots and bubbles can be discovered by pressure sensors in the instrument probes during analysis. Automated devices centrifuge, aliquot, and label aliquots based on the specimen barcode.

POSTANALYTICAL ERRORS

Reviewing data visually, in tables or text, is complicated. Reviewing results incorrectly can affect outcomes. Laboratorians and clinicians have different needs for data review within an electronic information system. Laboratory staff focus on individual test results and comments, while clinicians look for data trends in multiple analytes over time. Electronic information systems can display all test results chronologically, but data can also be displayed in a tabular form where test results for the same analyte are shown over time. Trends in results can more easily be followed in a tabular display across a row compared to scrolling through multiple pages of chronologically displayed full text results. However, there is no perfect means of displaying laboratory data. Viewing tables of numerical data poses a risk of loss of information. Clinicians want to review as much data on a single page or computer screen as possible, since this is more efficient than paging through multiple screens in the electronic record. Yet, cramming volumes of results in a table can risk loss of individual test comments and accompanying details with the potential for clinical misinterpretation if those comments contain significant information.

Errors in the transmission of data from the LIS to the physician can complicate analysis of test results. The display of test results for the ordering clinician is crucial to the clinical interpretation. The laboratory may think its role ends with the analysis and verification of a test result in the LIS, but physicians do not review test results in the LIS. Results must be transmitted to an electronic media record (EMR) for the physician to see the result. Glitches can occur in the communication interface between the LIS and the EMR that can change the result, trim the comments, or otherwise alter the test result and lead to errors.

How a test result is displayed can impact test interpretation. The recent push for ultrasensitive or third-generation assays emphasizes the clinical desire for higher sensitivity for disease detection. While an analyzer may be capable of reporting to a hundredth decimal place, the question is whether the method performance can achieve precision at that level to make the hundredth decimal point number meaningful. Reporting a result to two significant figures can mislead a clinician to assume better performance than can be achieved by the test method.

Results can be changed during transmission over electronic interfaces. The integrity of data transmission needs to be verified on an ongoing basis to ensure correct appearance for the ordering physician. Errors can occur when data are inadvertently changed as results are transmitted over electronic interfaces, with an obvious potential for result misinterpretation.

Managing access to information systems can be complicated and presents a source for potential duplicative analysis and errors. Information services can assist laboratory operations, particularly for the reporting of results to affiliated and nonaffiliated physician practices. While a goal of the EMR is to provide easy access to patient information as patients move throughout a health system (from inpatient to outpatient and to home health care), the stewards of the EMR also have the responsibility to protect the confidentiality of patient results and limit access to only those clinicians involved in the patient's care. The Health Insurance Portability and Accountability Act (HIPAA) of 1996 contains privacy regulations governing appropriate access to patient information. Determining and enforcing appropriate access to the EMR can be complicated, since patients may be seen at multiple sites, sometimes by physicians with competing clinical practices. Patients may seek advice from another physician in the form of a second opinion. Test results and medical record notes made by one physician should not necessarily be accessible to other physicians unless the results and records are released by the ordering physician or access is granted by the patient.

STANDARDS OF CARE

▓ Test names can be confusing and laboratories must distinguish tests of similar names according to their clinical application, methodology, limitations, or other unique characteristics.

▓ Electronic ordering systems must facilitate physician ordering of the appropriate tests, while limiting the ability of physicians to bypass the system or continue to use written requisitions.

▓ Staff must check at least two unique patient identifiers with any patient interaction, particularly for patients with common or similar-sounding names, and staff should heed electronic system warnings that are intended to catch certain identification errors.

▓ Presentation of laboratory data for clinician review must be easily understood. Tests results can be displayed in tabular form in an EMR to show more results on a single screen and improve efficiency of review, but more data come with the risk of losing individual result comments or specimen details and the associated potential for clinical misinterpretation. Requiring staff to actively seek out specimen comments rather than passively displaying information with the result poses the risk that the staff will miss clinically significant details. Laboratories should use an information system that draws attention easily to important details, rather than making users work to find the information.

While a goal of the EMR is to provide easy access to patient information as patients move throughout a health system (from inpatient to outpatient and home health care), stewards of the EMR must protect the confidentiality of patient results and limit access to only those clinicians involved in the patient's care.

Laboratory staff must be involved in the verification process of electronic data interfaces, since they can pose real-life situations that will challenge the reliability of the interface. Once implemented, interfaces require ongoing monitoring to ensure consistent display of data, as minor changes and updates to an information system can lead to unintended interface issues.

LABORATORY SAFETY

Safety is a key component of good laboratory practice and mandatory to permit basic operations to occur. Accidents occur because of unsafe workplace conditions. A first step to preventing accidents is to avoid unsafe conditions. The Occupational Safety and Health Administration (OSHA) is a federal agency concerned with employee safety and protection of employees from workplace injuries. OSHA enforces a number of federal regulations to ensure on-the-job safety for employees of all workplaces, not just the laboratory. A clinical laboratory presents particular hazards including exposure to patient specimens (e.g., with potential contact with infectious diseases and organisms), chemicals, electrical risks from laboratory instruments, and needle exposures. An employee can be injured simply by moving heavy instrumentation or boxes of supplies. Phlebotomists can suffer puncture injury during specimen collection. Service representatives can be injured during analyzer maintenance and repair. Couriers driving specimens between physician offices and the laboratory can be hurt from accidents in vehicles and even slips or falls in icy and wet conditions. Specimen processors that utilize high-speed centrifuges to spin tubes and separate the cellular components of blood can present a danger of flying metal, tube breakage, and specimen aerosols when operated incorrectly or with equipment failure. Technologists can contact corrosive acids and bases, and be exposed to fumes from volatile solvents when preparing reagents. There are a significant number of potential safety hazards in a clinical laboratory.

Administration also needs to consider the potential for injury to others beyond their laboratory employees. Improper disposal of chemicals down drains and common sewer lines can contaminate water sources such as ponds, lakes, and drinking water reservoirs, as well as presenting other environmental hazards. Failure to clean portable laboratory analyzers between patients when testing at the point-of-care presents a risk of transmitting hepatitis, HIV, or nosocomial infections among patients. Thus, safe laboratory operations consider all sources and effects of potential harm to employees, patients, the general public, and the environment.

PREANALYTICAL ERRORS

Food Risks

Eating and drinking in locations where laboratory tests are performed can affect both the test result and the person performing the test. A first commandment of today's laboratory safety is prohibiting eating and drinking in the laboratory. When specimens are being processed, the opening and aliquoting of tubes and specimen containers present a risk of aerosols, spills, splashes, and other sources of contamination of food and drink. While this principle may now seem common sense to laboratory technologists, managers, and directors, the hazards may not be so apparent when laboratory testing is actually conducted at the point-of-care by nurses.

Specimens that are spilled or splashed on countertops during testing can present a hazard if the countertops are not sufficiently cleaned after use. The presence of organisms (some of which may be resistant to antibiotics) risks a spread of nosocomial infections unless devices, reagents, and supplies are thoroughly cleaned and disinfected between patients. Contamination on countertops can be picked up on gloves and on the bottoms of reagent vials or meters and carried to other surfaces if adequate disinfection is not conducted after testing. Protective pads and other absorbent materials on laboratory benches can help contain specimens, but may not completely prevent contact with surfaces underneath the pad. Eating and drinking using the same surface where testing is conducted present a risk to staff and others consuming the food.

Failure to separate items intended for patient or employee use from laboratory specimens and supplies related to testing can cause problems. Consideration should be made for separation of clean linens, medications, and other supplies that could become contaminated in areas where laboratory testing is taking place. Food and medications that are intended for patient or employee consumption should not be stored in the same refrigerators as patient specimens or with potentially biohazardous controls or reagents made from blood products. Separate clean and dirty refrigerators are recommended and should be clearly labeled as to their intended purpose. Likewise, food served in patient care areas requires consideration for separation of areas that are potentially infectious from clean areas.

Chemical Hazards

Failure to ensure safe handling and storage of chemicals can be extremely dangerous. Safe laboratory operations require awareness of chemical hazards. Fumes from volatile chemicals can fill closed spaces and overwhelm staff. Such chemicals should be stored in vented cabinets and only utilized in fume hoods or rooms with adequate air exchange. Other chemicals can be hazardous when mixed, such as acids and bases. Metallic elements can become explosive in the presence of water. Laboratories need to carefully inventory the chemicals stored and utilized in their tests, provide for appropriate storage conditions, and ensure proper disposal.

Transportation and Processing

Specimen storage and transport can present hazardous situations. Couriers who transport specimens need to be concerned about the potential for container breakage and specimens leaking into cars or vans. The potential for a vehicle accident requires consideration that specimens could be released into the environment and contaminate surroundings. Specimens could be blood or body fluids containing agents for hepatitis or other bloodborne diseases, or, in a worst-case scenario, rare highly infectious pathogens destined for identification at state laboratories or the Centers for Disease Control and Prevention. This is why the Department of Transportation (DOT), the International Air Transport Association (IATA), and other agencies have enacted packaging and shipping regulations intended to contain specimens, even if they break in transit, to protect employees, the environment, and the general public from exposure during transit.

Laboratory instrumentation can present a safety hazard. Automated analyzers have a number of moving parts, and performing repairs and maintenance on working analyzers can lead to operator injury. Staff can be cut or punctured by moving probes, suffer electrical shock if they come into contact with the instrument after water leaks into the circuitry of the instrument, and be exposed to chemicals and body fluids if protective covers are moved during operation. Every area of the laboratory presents a safety risk if policies and procedures are not implemented to alert employees to the potential for harm. Staff should never run equipment without sufficient training, and should always take precautions to ensure appropriate operation whenever working with laboratory equipment.

STANDARDS OF CARE

▨ Staff should be cognizant of infection-control policies, the potential for surface contamination, and the need for routine cleaning and disinfection.

▨ DOT and IATA safety and shipping regulations must be enforced to protect employees handling specimens, the environment, and the general public from exposure to biohazardous pathogens.

▨ Personal protective equipment, that is, gloves, lab coat, safety glasses, and splash shields, must be used appropriately to protect staff from potential exposure to blood or fluids during specimen manipulation.

▨ There must be separation of clean supplies, such as linens, medications, and medical equipment, from areas where laboratory testing is taking place.

▨ Surfaces, such as countertops, medical equipment, testing devices, beds, railings, and nightstands, can become contaminated with antibiotic-resistant organisms and require regular cleaning and disinfection, especially when shared between patients.

▨ Chemicals that present a risk of fire, fumes, burns, or other safety concerns for staff require handling, storage, and disposal according to specific guidelines.

▨ Staff should never run equipment without training and should always take precautions to ensure appropriate operation whenever working with laboratory equipment.

OUTREACH TESTING

Outreach testing is an extension of a hospital laboratory to test samples from outside the institution, such as the region around the laboratory, including from private physician office practices, other hospitals, long-term care facilities, and other sites. Increasing the outpatient volume of samples increases laboratory profitability, since insurance companies currently pay for laboratory tests as a fee for service on a per-test basis for outpatient visits. In contrast, there is a single flat reimbursement for inpatients for all costs incurred based on a diagnosis that encompasses the entire treatment. Thus, many hospitals are seeking to expand their laboratory testing market by partnering with local physician offices. Outreach testing programs are a growing business model as health care finances get tighter.

The outreach business model provides advantages for both parties. Physicians will have access to local expertise in the laboratory, while the hospital receives the additional sample volume. Physician offices find local laboratories more accessible, and on that basis, more responsive to inquiries, as compared with national reference laboratories that may have automated answering machines and may require multiple transfers to reach someone who is knowledgeable enough to manage their question.

Unfortunately, an outreach business based on profit and client growth can sometimes be at odds with inpatient cost containment and test utilization strategies. Hospital laboratories engaging in outreach will need to invest in a sales and marketing staff, which was not a consideration prior to outreach. At least some of the sales staff may have never worked in a laboratory and may not realize the medical applications of specific tests or method limitations and interferences. Their job is to satisfy clients and provide better service than the national reference laboratories against whom they are competing. While medical directors may be ensuring that inpatient physicians order the right test for a specific patient's suspected condition and limit test overutilization, outreach sales personnel are promoting physician ordering and inadvertently, or otherwise, overordering. For outreach work, there is emphasis on the old business adage that the client is always right. While medical directors may seek to limit or place an "approval-only ordering" rule on certain high-cost esoteric tests for inpatients, the goal of outreach sales is to facilitate their clients' ability to get any test to keep the account. Conflicts can arise when physicians can freely order esoteric and routine tests for their office patients, but are limited and restricted from ordering the same tests on their inpatients. This dynamic creates the potential for laboratory miscommunication, conflict, and errors. While standardization across the system may be best, budgets and politics may limit a laboratory's ability to implement one-size-fits-all policies across all inpatient, outpatient, and outreach operations.

PREANALYTICAL ERRORS

Communication breakdowns between laboratory operation teams and other departments can cause serious problems. Common policies and procedures should be the goal throughout an organization. However, outreach programs are often managed by business managers, while inpatient laboratory operations are more directly supervised by medical directors. This creates two separate business operations within the laboratory, sometimes with different and conflicting goals and policies. Problems can occur when communication breaks down between the two operations, and the outreach managers develop policies and procedures independent of existing laboratory operations.

Even minor changes in clinical testing procedures can have a serious effect on patient outcomes. Medical director participation in the management of hospital outreach programs is required to adequately recognize and prevent certain errors. Medical directors have a perspective on the clinical utilization of test results as well as preanalytical sources of error that sales and administrative staff in hospital outreach programs may not appreciate. What may seem to be a minor change in practice could lead to significant effects on patient results. Operational changes should be routinely reviewed by a medical director for potential issues.

When a lab has to involve another lab to get complete test results and there is a different quality of customer service between the labs, physicians can have unsatisfactory experiences. A laboratory is sometimes the consumer rather than the provider of laboratory testing. No single laboratory can perform all possible tests that could be ordered by hospital staff or physician offices. At one time or another, every laboratory must send a sample to another laboratory for analysis. This may occur because the volume of a particular test is low, the test requires specialized equipment or staffing, or the test is so esoteric that the laboratory simply cannot set up the test. Certain tests are also proprietary and are only performed by one laboratory. As a consumer of laboratory tests, clinical staff can get a different impression of customer service offered by a laboratory because the test requested is actually performed by a different laboratory. Difficulties reaching someone who can answer a question or inconsistencies in results between outside laboratories can leave the physician with a poor impression of laboratory quality.

POSTANALYTICAL ERRORS

The complexity of multiple laboratories performing and billing for specimen analysis can be confusing to physicians and patients. The laboratory performing a test is generally responsible for billing the patient's insurance. If the insurance company does not cover the costs of the test or only partially reimburses, then the patient may be responsible for the difference. Therefore, the patient may receive a bill from both the physician's office for a visit, and a separate bill from the laboratory for tests associated with that visit. When a hospital laboratory cannot perform the requested test and the specimen is sent to a referral laboratory, the hospital laboratory may receive the bill from the referral laboratory directly. The hospital laboratory is then responsible for billing and recovering the referral laboratory charges from either the patient's insurance or the patient directly. If neither pays, then the hospital laboratory suffers the loss. Some reference laboratories will directly bill the patient's insurance ("third-party billing") and will take on the financial risk if the insurance or patient does not pay. In such cases, patients may receive a bill for test results from an unfamiliar laboratory.

Timely reporting of test results can be challenging. Laboratories have the responsibility for timely reporting of test results to outreach clients, just as they would for their own hospitalized inpatients. Unfortunately, many outreach clients are physician offices that are closed after hours. These physician offices may have intermittent coverage that can present a challenge to laboratories that need to reach the ordering physician after hours.

STANDARDS OF CARE

▧ Laboratory outreach expands the current laboratory operations beyond the walls of the hospital, but uniform policies and procedures must be in place to ensure comparable quality of testing.
▧ A New Technology Committee provides a forum for stakeholders to review the advantages, limitations, and financial consequences of using a new product or laboratory test. Such a committee should

be implemented to develop consensus decisions for new technology, including laboratory testing.

▓ Ordering physicians have the responsibility to discuss the benefits and limitations of diagnostic testing with patients.

▓ A laboratory must inform physicians to make them up-to-date with current testing trends, costs, and the menu of tests performed internally as well as the tests referred to other laboratories.

▓ A critical result is a laboratory value that represents an imminently life-threatening clinical situation and requires immediate communication to a physician. The laboratory must contact a clinician in real time, either the ordering physician or their designee who can take clinical action, to communicate a critical result and verify accurate understanding of the communication via read-back. Hospital outreach is a business model for expanding laboratory services that require sales and marketing administration, but clinical and technical oversight of the operation also requires medical director participation.

▓ Hospital outreach that facilitates any test that a physician wants may sometimes be at odds with hospital laboratory goals of limiting test utilization. Communication is essential between outreach sales staff who may have little laboratory experience and the laboratory staff and medical directors with extensive clinical and technical experience.

BIBLIOGRAPHY

Clinical and Laboratory Standards Institute. *EP23-A: Laboratory Quality Control Based on Risk Management; Approved Guideline*. Wayne, PA: Clinical and Laboratory Standards Institute; 2011.

College of American Pathologists Laboratory Accreditation Program. *Chemistry and Toxicology Checklist*. Northfield, IL: CAP; 2012.

College of American Pathologists Laboratory Accreditation Program. *Point-of-Care Testing Checklist*. Northfield, IL: College of American Pathologists; 2012.

Department of Health and Human Services Health Care Financing Administration Public Health Service 42 CFR. Final rule: Medicare, Medicaid, and CLIA programs. Regulations implementing Clinical Laboratories Improvement Amendments of 1988 (CLIA). *Fed Regist*. 1992;57:7001–7288.

International Air Transport Association. *Dangerous Goods Regulations Manual*. 54th ed. Geneva, Switzerland: International Air Transport Association; 2013.

Joint Commission. *2013 CAMLAB: Comprehensive Accreditation Manual Laboratory and Point-of-Care Testing*. Oakbrook, IL: The Joint Commission; 2013.

National Academy of Clinical Biochemistry. *Laboratory Medicine Practice Guidelines; Evidence-Based Practice for Point-of-Care Testing*. Washington, DC: AACC Press; 2006.

National Academy of Clinical Biochemistry. *Laboratory Medicine Practice Guidelines. Laboratory Support for the Diagnosis and Monitoring of Thyroid Disease*. Washington, DC: AACC Press; 2002.

NCCLS. *H21-A4: Collection, Transport, and Processing of Blood Specimens for Testing Plasma-Based Coagulation Assays: Approved Guideline*. 4th ed. Wayne, PA: NCCLS; 2003:23.

U.S. Pipeline and Hazardous Materials Safety Administration, Department of Transportation. Code of federal regulations, subchapter C, hazardous materials regulations. CFR 49, Part 171–173. October 1, 2011.

CHAPTER 5
Clinical Microbiology

CHARLES W. STRATTON

Clinical microbiologists are well aware of the adage
first coined by computer programmers, "garbage in,
garbage out," but for their profession have renamed it
"quality in, quality out." Their adage refers to the fact
that the quality of the clinical specimen received by the
clinical microbiology laboratory is a key factor in the
optimal use of clinical microbiology. For serological
testing, the timing of the serum collection may be an
equally critical factor for optimal use. Unfortunately,
the clinicians often do not have the tools, interest,
training, access to data, or time to determine optimal
use of the clinical microbiology laboratory for their
patients. This chapter discusses common preanalytic
medical errors in the clinical microbiology laboratory.

FAILURE TO CONSIDER INFECTION

*Failure to consider infection is actually a more common
problem than one might think. It seems to center around
surgical procedures where a malignancy is suspected. Thus,
oncologists and surgeons must be alert and always consider
the possibility of infection even when malignancy is their
first concern.*

Not sending material from a clinical specimen to the clinical microbiology laboratory for culture or other microbiological testing may result in this type of preanalytic medical error. This is a very subtle type of medical error and is considered an individual type of error that is not easily rectified by a systems approach. Bone marrow aspirations and biopsies are often done to rule out malignancy; cultures may not be requested on the aspirate/biopsy as the clinicians are focused on malignancy and not thinking about infection. Oncologists and surgeons must be alert and always consider the possibility of infection even when malignancy is their first concern.

For example, failure to consider infection may occur when evaluating a patient with neck mass and/or cervical lymphadenopathy in which lymphoma or metastatic carcinoma is the working diagnosis. Because lymph node biopsy is often reserved for situations in which a malignant process is suspected, the clinician may not think to order cultures. Biopsy for asymptomatic cervical lymphadenopathy of greater than three weeks' duration is a common situation in which metastatic carcinoma is suspected, particularly in patients over 40 years of age. These enlarged cervical lymph nodes thus are usually excised or biopsied, and the lymphatic tissue is sent to the surgical pathology laboratory. If cultures are desired, the surgeon must send part of the lymphatic tissue to the clinical microbiology laboratory. Lymphatic tissue sent to the surgical pathology laboratory is fixed in formalin, which precludes additional tests such as tissue cultures when the hematoxylin and eosin (H&E) examination reveals lymphadenitis. Failure to send part of the lymphatic tissue to the clinical microbiology laboratory for culture is a particular problem in children, in whom nontuberculous cervical lymphadenopathy is more commonly seen. Infections that may present with cervical lymphadenopathy include cervical mycobacterial infections (*Mycobacterium tuberculosis* [MTB] and *Mycobacterium avian* complex), cat scratch disease (*Bartonella henselae*), histoplasmosis, and toxoplasmosis.

Biopsy of indeterminate mediastinal masses, which is often done in order to evaluate the mediastinal mass/lymph nodes for malignancy, presents another example. When histopathologic examination reveals no malignancy, the opportunity for culture has passed. The demonstration of microorganisms by special stains may provide the diagnosis. Tuberculosis is an unusual cause of mediastinal mass in an infant, but in contrast, histoplasmosis as a cause of mediastinal mass in an infant or in a child has been reported on many occasions. These cases of mediastinal histoplasmosis in children were sometimes mistakenly diagnosed as lymphoma. There is a significant risk for medical errors in cases involving a mediastinal mass in a child if infection is not considered.

Lung infections mimicking malignancy are another relevant presentation that is well described in the medical literature. An important reason for this is that both pulmonary infections and pulmonary malignancies are initially detected by a radiologic diagnostic procedure such as a chest radiograph x-ray or a chest computed tomography scan. Radiologic features suggestive of a pulmonary malignancy include a parenchymal mass with speculated margins, microlobulations, thick-walled cavity, cavity showing nodular margins, and chest wall invasion. These findings, however, are not specific and can be seen with pulmonary infections. If the possibility of an infection is not considered, the diagnostic procedures done may not include those measures such as culture that are necessary to detect infection. In one large series of over 2,000 patients who underwent a lung biopsy with a presumed diagnosis of malignancy, 37 (1.3%) of these cases were found to have infection rather than malignancy. Fungal infections accounted for 46% of the infections diagnosed in this series. Thus, the clinician must keep in mind the possibility of infection when initiating diagnostic procedures to confirm a presumed pulmonary malignancy.

STANDARDS OF CARE

▪ Failure to consider infection can result in a medical error when material from biopsy specimens is not sent to the clinical microbiology laboratory because malignancy is considered the most likely diagnosis; when the tissue turns out to not be malignant, the lack of a culture result may result in harm to the patient.

▪ Conversely, sending material for culture from a tissue biopsy specimen that ultimately turns out to be malignant is not considered a medical error; the culture will not grow and no harm to the patient will result.

▪ Oncologists and surgeons, in particular, must remember that infections are able to mimic malignancy; therefore, obtaining cultures of biopsy tissues should be carefully considered when biopsies are being done to rule out or confirm suspected cancer.

FAILURE TO CONSIDER UNCOMMON INFECTIONS

Failure to consider uncommon infections is another common medical error seen in infectious diseases and clinical microbiology. This type of error is best avoided by obtaining consultation (informal or formal) from infectious disease clinicians and/or the clinical microbiology laboratory director.

Consider the example of failure to consider an uncommon infection such as ehrlichiosis/anaplasmosis in the differential diagnosis of a febrile patient with "summer flu." This error may, at best, delay the diagnosis of this infection, which can cause significant morbidity and mortality if not suspected and treated promptly. Recognition of ehrlichiosis/anaplasmosis as a possible diagnosis requires the treating clinician to have knowledge about tickborne illnesses, which are an emerging infectious threat. Alternatively, consultation with an infectious diseases clinician may avoid such a medical error. Serologic testing does not usually help in the diagnosis of acute ehrlichiosis, as seroconversion may not occur until three weeks into the illness. Treatment thus should be initiated based on the clinical presentation and not based on the results of laboratory testing. A polymerase chain reaction (PCR) assay for ehrlichiosis is an alternative method for diagnosing this illness and is more likely to be positive. The availability of a PCR assay for ehrlichiosis depends on the capabilities of an individual clinical microbiology laboratory. Even if the PCR assay is available, treatment for ehrlichiosis should be initiated before the PCR result is available. Finally, making a PCR assay for ehrlichiosis available for a more rapid diagnosis may require costly upgrading of the molecular diagnostic capabilities of the clinical microbiology laboratory.

Another uncommon infection is Rocky Mountain spotted fever (RMSF), which is similar to ehrlichiosis/anaplasmosis in a number of ways. In both cases, initial failure to consider a tickborne illness in summer months can result in a delay in the diagnosis and treatment of an infection. With RMSF, a potential outcome is rickettsial meningoencephalitis resulting in death. RMSF is still the most lethal tickborne illness in the United States. Pitfalls related to the evaluation of the patient with possible RMSF include (a) waiting for the rash to develop, (b) misdiagnosing the febrile illness as another infection such as gastroenteritis, (c) discounting the diagnosis in the absence of history of tick bite, (d) using an inappropriate geographic exclusion, (e) using an inappropriate seasonal exclusion, (f) failing to treat on clinical suspicion, (g) failing to elicit an appropriate history, and (h) failing to treat with doxycycline. The diagnosis of RMSF has been, and continues to be, problematic. The most widely used diagnostic tool is serologic testing, which is not useful during active infection. Seroconversion of RMSF infection may not occur until three weeks into the illness. PCR assays for diagnosing RMSF have been developed, but to date these assays have not been fully evaluated in the clinical setting. A critical issue in their usefulness would be the length of time that *Rickettsia rickettsii* would remain in the blood. Combined PCR and electrospray ionization mass spectrometry method may be able to detect both *Ehrlichia* species and *R. rickettsii*. The diagnosis and empirical doxycycline therapy of RMSF is particularly difficult in children as pediatricians, family physicians, and/or emergency room physicians may not appreciate that RMSF is seen in children or be aware that the appropriate treatment strategy requires doxycycline treatment before the rash is seen. Finally, it should be noted that a newly recognized tickborne spotted fever group rickettsiosis has been described. The cause of this tickborne escar-associated spotted fever group rickettsiosis is *Rickettsia parkeri*, which originally was thought to be nonpathogenic in humans. Clinically, this rickettsiosis presents in a manner that is very similar to RMSF with symptoms of fever, fatigue, myalgia, headache, and a generalized rash; in addition, patients describe a "sore" or "pimple" at the site of a tick bite. This escar typically precedes the onset of fever by several days. This illness, like RMSF, is mostly seen in the southeastern Unites States. As with RMSF, empirical therapy with doxycycline should be initiated in patients with this constellation of symptoms.

Babesiosis is another tickborne infection seen during summer months that can be particularly difficult to identify unless it is considered in the differential diagnosis. Clinically, babesiosis resembles malaria and is endogenous to the United States. Observing intraerythrocytic ring-forms in a blood smear can quickly make the diagnosis if the clinician requests such smears. Otherwise, multiple episodes of a febrile illness may go undiagnosed until a routine blood smear and/or an alert medical technologist allow the diagnosis of babesiosis to be made. Patients may require the review of multiple thin and thick blood smears to make a diagnosis. Diagnosis may be made serendipitously on a routine blood smear; however, autoanalyzers or a less observant medical technologist might miss this diagnosis, and multiple blood smears and/

or thick smears may be required. A careful review by a medical technologist or pathologist of abnormal red blood cell images stored in current blood autoanalyzers is the best way to make a diagnosis of babesiosis, as there are far more red blood cells screened and abnormal red blood cells stored as an image than is possible with a blood smear. Finally, PCR methods have been described, but are not widely available. Moreover, the diagnosis must be considered before a PCR assay can be ordered.

Lyme disease represents another case in which failure to consider an uncommon tickborne infection may lead to diagnostic confusion. Tickborne infections should be considered in the differential diagnosis for a febrile illness in a patient with thrombocytopenia, especially in a patient presenting in summer. Early Lyme disease is particularly difficult to diagnose and empirical antimicrobial therapy should be considered with the appropriate clinical situation. Antigenic stimulus due to *Borrelia burgdorferi* infection is known to cause a blastoid transformation of B and T lymphocytes that can result in cerebrospinal fluid (CSF) cytology mimicking central nervous system malignancy.

STANDARDS OF CARE

▓ Failure to consider uncommon infections clearly can result in harm to a patient; it may be less clear that a medical error has occurred although the patient and/or a lawyer would likely consider such a failure to be a medical error.

▓ Failure to consider uncommon infections as a source of medical errors can be avoided by a number of mechanisms; these include use of the medical literature, use of the Internet (e.g., PubMed or *UpToDate*), consultation with the clinical microbiology laboratory director, and consultation with an infectious diseases clinician.

▓ Tickborne infections are an emerging infectious threat and cause uncommon infections that must be considered in the differential diagnosis of febrile patients seen during summer months in order to avoid medical errors.

▓ Broad-spectrum empirical antimicrobial therapy may be needed while the differential diagnosis is being developed and the results of diagnostic testing are pending; this is particularly true for tickborne infections where only babesiosis can be quickly diagnosed.

FAILURE TO APPRECIATE THE PROPER TIMING FOR SEROLOGY TESTS

Failure to appreciate the proper timing for serology is another common medical error and leads to confusion when the "obvious" diagnosis is "ruled out" by the serologic test. Consultation with the laboratory can assist with this problem.

Acute West Nile encephalitis presents a case illustrating the need for proper timing of serologic testing. Acute West Nile encephalitis is a serious public health issue in the United States with over 700 cases reported to the Centers for Disease Control and Prevention (CDC) in 2009. The CDC recommends that West Nile virus immunoglobulin M (IgM) detection by an IgM capture enzyme-linked immunosorbent assay (ELISA) in serum or CSF should be the major laboratory tool used to identify symptomatic patients with acute West Nile virus infections. This test has a sensitivity approaching 100% in appropriately timed samples. In early symptomatic infections, the West Nile virus can be detected by PCR in serum or CSF. However, levels of West Nile virus RNA typically peak before symptoms appear and then rapidly decline as IgM antibody production begins. Thus, there is a limited window for RNA detection. Once IgM antibodies for West Nile virus appear, they remain detectable for several months after the acute illness. Although most patients with West Nile virus encephalitis present late in their illness, some patients seeking medical assistance within a week of symptom onset may still be in the RNA-positive/antibody-negative window and the infection may be missed if only IgM testing is done. To avoid missing cases of acute West Nile infection, both West Nile virus RNA testing and West Nile virus IgM testing may be required. However, as there is no current antiviral therapy for West Nile virus encephalitis, a delay in the diagnosis may not present a therapeutic problem.

Proper timing is also relevant in the serologic diagnosis of Lyme disease. Serology may not allow the diagnosis of early Lyme disease. Suspicion of Lyme disease based on erythema migrans is sufficient reason to begin empiric antimicrobial therapy.

Leptospirosis presents another infection where the timing of testing is relevant. Leptospirosis is a zoonotic disease caused by the spirochetes of the genus *Leptospira* and is considered to be one of the most common zoonoses in the world. In the past decade, leptospirosis has been recognized as an emerging public health problem that occurs in urban and rural areas of developing and developed countries. Humans are accidental hosts and become infected through exposure to environmental sources contaminated by the urine of chronically infected mammals. In the United States, the most common sources of exposure are dogs, livestock, and wild animals, especially rodents. Outbreaks of leptospirosis have been reported and are often due to natural disasters such as floods. Leptospirosis is also recognized as an infection seen in travelers returning from the tropics. Patients hospitalized with leptospirosis may have mortality rates as high as 25%; this is, in part, related to a delay in diagnosis. The majority of leptospirosis cases are diagnosed by serology. The current standard is the microscopic agglutination test, which involves the reaction of antigens in the form of live *Leptospira* organisms with the antibodies found in the patient's sera. A positive reaction results in agglutination of the *Leptospira* that can be seen microscopically. The IgG antibody response to leptospirosis for this test takes about two weeks and can be delayed by antimicrobial therapy. New serologic methods are commercially available; some of these tests measure an IgM response and may thus allow more rapid results. PCR testing is also being developed and should allow the most rapid means of diagnosis.

STANDARDS OF CARE

■ Certain infectious diseases such as many viral infections, as well as infections involving *Mycoplasma*, *Leptospira*, *Borrelia*, *Treponema*, *Coxiella*, and *Chlamydia*, often require a serologic diagnosis; appreciation of the time required for an antibody response to the acute infection is important when obtaining such serologic tests.

■ Failure to appreciate the proper timing for serology tests can result in harm to a patient even though the correct diagnosis was considered, and an appropriate serology test was ordered; failure to appreciate the proper timing for serology tests is a subtle but real form of medical error.

■ Unlike failure to consider infection or failure to consider uncommon infections, in this situation the correct infection was considered; using empirical antimicrobial therapy when applicable can avoid this type of medical error.

■ Appreciating the appropriate timing of serology tests may result in repeating a serology test that is initially negative; empirical antimicrobial therapy as mentioned earlier prevents harm to the patient.

FAILURE TO APPRECIATE THE SENSITIVITY OR SPECIFICITY OF MICROBIOLOGY TESTS

Failure to appreciate the sensitivity or specificity of microbiology tests is another common problem and can lead to medical errors. This problem often can be avoided by consultation with the laboratory.

The need to understand the sensitivity and specificity of specific microbiology tests was illustrated vividly during the spring and summer of 2009, when a novel influenza A virus of swine origin, H1N1, emerged in humans in North America. The sensitivity of rapid diagnostic tests for influenza during the peak influenza season is approximately 60%; a lower prevalence of influenza at other times of the year will result in a lower sensitivity for rapid influenza testing. Nasopharyngeal swabs are preferred over buccal swabs. Empiric antiviral treatment should be based on the clinical picture rather than the results of rapid influenza testing. The Infectious Diseases Society of America Clinical Practice Guidelines currently recommend early treatment (ideally within 48 hours) with oseltamivir or zanamivir for persons in whom influenza virus infection is highly suspected. Unfortunately, such treatments were not recommended by the CDC in early summer of 2009.

Cryptococcal meningitis is another case where use of a sensitive culture method is critical to accurate diagnosis. Cryptococcal antigen and crytococcal CSF cultures are both of limited value, and BACTEC Myco/F Lytic bottle is more sensitive. In particular, capsule-deficient isolates of *Cryptococcus neoformans* are known to cause difficulty in diagnosing chronic cryptococcal meningitis using the CSF cryptococcal latex agglutination test. In nonimmunosuppressed patients, the delayed diagnosis of cryptococcal meningitis is a recognized problem that has increased the morbidity and mortality of this condition. False-positive cryptococcal antigen testing has been reported and must be considered in such antigen testing.

Diagnosis of *Legionella* infection is also limited by the nonspecific nature of clinical features and the shortcomings of diagnostic tests. *Legionella* species are important causes of pneumonia in humans. Currently, of the more than 50 species of *Legionella,* at least 24 are associated with human disease. Although *Legionella pneumophila* appears to be more pathogenic to humans and causes the majority of human disease, other species clearly can infect humans. Importantly, cavitary pulmonary infection has been associated with *Legionella bozemanii*. *Legionella micdadei* and *Legionella longbeachae* are other common etiologic agents causing human infection. Unfortunately, no single microbiology test is able to diagnose *Legionella* infection in a timely fashion with a high degree of sensitivity and specificity. Although *Legionella* culture remains the most useful single test, culture diagnosis requires special media, adequate processing of specimens, and technical expertise. The standard medium used to culture *Legionella* species is buffered charcoal yeast extract (BCYE) agar. Supplementation of BCYE agar with bovine serum albumin will enhance the growth of some *Legionella* species such as *L. bozemanii* and *L. micdadei*; in contrast, addition of cefamandole to this agar, as is often done, will inhibit growth of these two species. Despite the appropriate use of BCYE agar for sputum cultures, the sensitivity of expectorated sputum cultures ranges from 10% to 80% as fewer than half of patients with *Legionella* pneumonia produce sputum. Bronchoscopy or pulmonary biopsy specimens are more likely to yield positive cultures than are expectorated sputum samples. The detection of soluble *Legionella* antigen in urine specimens has become a rapid and reliable tool for the diagnosis of *L. pneumophila* infections. These urinary antigen tests have sensitivities in the range of 70% to 100% but are only able to detect *L. pneumophila* serogroup 1. Other species of *Legionella* are not reliably detected. False-positive results for the *Legionella* urinary antigen have been reported as well. Serologic testing for *Legionella* infection is hampered by the delay in seroconversion, which may take several weeks, as well as by the inability of serologic testing to accurately detect all *Legionella* species and subgroups. Clearly, there remains a role for *Legionella* cultures obtained by bronchoscopy or pulmonary biopsy.

STANDARDS OF CARE

▨ Failure to appreciate the sensitivity or specificity of microbiology tests can result in harm to a patient even though the correct diagnosis was considered, and an appropriate microbiology test was ordered; failure to appreciate the sensitivity or specificity of microbiology tests is a subtle but real form of medical error.

▨ The sensitivity and specificity of antigen testing in clinical microbiology is particularly important; both false-negative and false-positive test results are factors in such antigen testing and must be appreciated.

▨ Consultations with the clinical microbiology laboratory and/ or the infectious diseases unit are excellent ways to avoid this potential error.

FAILURE TO SUBMIT A SUITABLE MICROBIOLOGY SPECIMEN

Failure to submit suitable microbiology specimens is unfortunately a common problem that can lead to medical errors in infectious diseases and clinical microbiology. Consultation with the clinical microbiology laboratory regarding suitable specimens is the best way to avoid this error.

Skin and soft tissue abscesses present an area where suitable specimen collection may be crucial. Areas of debate here include the usefulness of cultures and empiric treatment with antimicrobial agents. The increasing incidence of community-associated methicillin-resistant staphylococcus aureus (CA-MRSA) has intensified this debate. *Nocardia* species, for instance, often take five days or longer to grow on sheep blood agar, so a "no growth" culture result after 48 hours would not assist in the care of such a patient. Holding the culture longer than two days may allow the diagnosis and appropriate therapy. If this infection is not diagnosed, the *Nocardia* infection may eventually progress to involve deeper tissues and bone in the foot; a type of infection known as "Madura foot," for example, is very difficult to treat and often leads to amputation of the infected foot.

The value of sputum Gram stain and culture in the diagnosis of community-acquired pneumonia is another area of considerable debate. Obtaining a good-quality sputum specimen is difficult in young, nonexpectorating children with pneumonia. Routine sputum collection and analysis has not been recommended in children with community-acquired pneumonia for a number of reasons. Among these cogent reasons are that viral pneumonia is the most common cause of community-acquired pneumonia during the first two years and that young children cannot easily expectorate sputum. Moreover, empiric therapy with newer cephalosporins generally has proven effective in situations in which clinicians suspect a bacterial cause of community-acquired pneumonia in a child. Resistance to newer cephalosporins can result in treatment failure leading to readmission to the hospital. Collection of sputum in children or in adults is likely to be very important in the near future when traditional diagnostic methods are supplemented with PCR-based methods in order to increase the microbiological yield for the etiology of community-acquired pneumonia.

Malaria evaluation is another case in which the failure to submit a suitable microbiology specimen may be problematic. Peripheral blood examinations performed using automated equipment may be inadequate. The number of fields scanned by a technologist on these smears using automated equipment is quite low, and thus failure to pick up a light malarial parasitemia is not unusual. More extensive scanning of the blood fields stored in automated blood equipment by a pathologist is, however, an excellent way to make a diagnosis of malaria. The initial key to the diagnosis of malaria is travel history (e.g., South America) as the incubation period can be variable for all strains of malaria. Indeed, fever in a returned traveler must always raise the possibility of malaria in the differential diagnosis.

In addition, imported malaria in visitors to the United States must also be considered in febrile patients with vague and nonspecific clinical presentations of malaria who may be seen in emergency rooms. Thin and thick smears for malaria should be ordered as the parasitemia may be missed with routine complete blood counts done on automated instruments. Thrombocytopenia is the most common laboratory abnormality encountered with malaria, seen in approximately 60% of cases regardless of the type of malaria, and should also prompt a blood smear. Hyperbilirubinemia is also seen in approximately 40% of malaria cases, and anemia is seen in approximately 30%. The presence of thrombocytopenia and hyperbilirubinemia alone has a positive predictive value of 95% in the presumptive diagnosis of malaria in the febrile traveler returning from a part of the world where malaria is endemic. It is important to understand that babesiosis can also present with fever, thrombocytopenia, hyperbilirubinemia, and anemia and also may require thin and thick blood smears for diagnosis; routine complete blood counts on automated instruments may miss this diagnosis for the same reason that malaria can be missed. Clearly, not sending blood for parasite analysis (i.e., malaria and babesiosis) can represent a failure to submit a suitable specimen in a febrile patient.

Mycotic infections provide yet another example of the importance of collecting suitable specimens. Chromoblastomycosis is a chronic mycotic infection caused by pigmented saprophytic molds of the Dermatiaceae family ubiquitous in the environment. The members of the Dermatiaceae family are dimorphic filamentous fungi with melanic-type pigment in the cell wall. Clinically, the infection usually follows traumatic inoculation through penetrating thorn or splinter wounds and is characterized by the development of chronic verrucose lesions at the inoculation site. *Phialophora richardsiae* is a recognized cause of chromoblastomycosis in humans and can cause osteomyelitis. Puncture wounds of the foot can result in serious complications such as osteomyelitis. For this reason, puncture wounds may require wound enlargement and a search for a retained foreign body. Imbedded rubber foreign bodies from footwear and thorn or wood splinters are recognized risk factors for infection. Biopsy with appropriate cultures should be done initially rather than relying on empiric antimicrobial therapy. Gram-negative bacteria such as *Pseudomonas aeruginosa* can cause osteomyelitis following puncture wounds of the foot. However, other microorganisms including fungi or mycobacteria can also cause osteomyelitis of the calcaneus secondary to a puncture wound. It thus is important to realize that when cultures are ordered in calcaneal osteomyelitis following a puncture wound, bacterial, fungal, and mycobacterial cultures should be specified on the requisition.

Infection with *Staphylococcus aureus* and MTB may also cause osteomyelitis. If bone cultures for *Mycobacterium* are not done, and granulomatous inflammation without demonstrable acid-fast bacilli is seen, there are two potential solutions. The first solution is to recut the formalin-fixed, paraffin-embedded tissue for additional acid-fast staining. Additional sections cut for acid-fast staining will sometimes identify acid-fast bacilli not seen in the first cuts. The second solution is to use molecular detection methods such as PCR testing for *M. tuberculosis*; these are done on the formalin-fixed, paraffin-embedded tissue, and have proven successful in such situations. Such testing is best done in consultation with the clinical microbiology laboratory. In general, bone specimens from patients with vertebral osteomyelitis should include bacterial, fungal, and mycobacterial cultures in order to avoid this type of medical error. Molecular testing is a reasonable adjunct test when mycobacterial cultures have not been done or are negative.

STANDARDS OF CARE

▨ Failure to submit a suitable microbiology specimen or any microbiology specimen at all even though infection is suspected may happen for a number of reasons and can be another subtle form of medical error.

- If unusual microorganisms are suspected, the clinical microbiology laboratory should be consulted as special media and/or incubating the cultures for a prolonged period of time might be necessary; such consultation may also result in assistance in terms of what type of cultures should be ordered on specimens from a febrile patient.

- Consultation with infectious diseases clinicians is also useful in determining what type of cultures should be obtained in a febrile patient.

- Fever in returning travelers or foreign travelers visiting the United States should raise the diagnostic possibility of malaria; thick and thin blood smears for malaria are indicated in this situation.

- Mixed infections with dissimilar microorganisms such as bacteria and fungi or bacteria and mycobacteria do occur; specimens sent to the clinical microbiology laboratory must specifically request bacterial, fungal, and mycobacterial cultures in order to ensure that all are done.

- Molecular diagnostic techniques now may offer a "second chance" to make the correct diagnosis if appropriate cultures are not requested on the specimen initially sent to the clinical microbiology laboratory.

- The pathophysiology of a suspected infection may provide insight on additional tissue that can be biopsied for culture and/or PCR testing when initial testing is nonrevealing.

FAILURE TO PROPERLY IDENTIFY PATIENT, SPECIMEN, OR TEST ORDER

Failure to properly identify patient, specimen, or test order is a common issue in all laboratories. Attention to detail and electronic bar code labeling can assist with this problem.

Rejection and recollection of a specimen once mislabeling is detected is the most suitable approach to managing this issue; that is, the microbiology technologist may call the emergency room so that the person who obtained a blood culture that appears mislabeled may come to the microbiology laboratory and properly label the bottles. This solution may not be possible, however, if antimicrobial agents have been initiated. An unlabeled blood culture bottle might appear to be a minor issue that is easily resolved, but this type of preanalytic phase medical error is extremely common and has great potential for becoming a major issue. Consider a case, for instance, in which there is more than one unlabeled set of blood culture bottles, each set from two separate patients. Assume also that these were received in the microbiology laboratory at the same time. Properly labeling these two sets of blood culture bottles would become a major problem.

The preanalytic phase of laboratory testing is manually intensive and thus prone to having the highest error rate. Blood collection is a particularly error-prone portion of the total laboratory testing process. Among the common preanalytic phase errors are mistakes in tube filling, inappropriate containers, inappropriate requesting procedures, and identification errors (i.e., misidentification). Indeed, misidentification has been identified as a major problem in the preanalytic phase of laboratory testing with the following causes being the most problematic: (a) physician ordering a laboratory test on the wrong patient, (b) incorrect or incomplete computer entry of patient's data, (c) collection of a specimen from the wrong patient, (d) inappropriate labeling of the specimen, (e) lost identification (label or requisition) for the specimen, and (f) incorrect entry of the patient's results in the computer database.

Clearly the preanalytic phase of laboratory testing is vulnerable to errors; most of these errors result from system flaws and insufficient audit and control of the operators involved in specimen collection. A number of factors must be considered in order to deal with these types of preanalytic errors. The first factor to consider is prediction of accidental events, which is accomplished by the following processes: (a) exhaustive process analysis, (b) reassessment and rearrangement of quality requirements, (c) dissemination of operating guidelines and best-practice recommendations, (d) reduction of complexity and error-prone activities, (e) introduction of error-tracking systems, (f) continuous monitoring of performance, and (g) root cause analysis of any errors identified to ensure that any systems flaws can be addressed.

The next factor to consider is an increase in and diversification of defenses, which is accomplished by the application of multiple and heterogeneous systems to identify nonconformities. The final factor to consider is a decrease in vulnerability, which is accomplished by implementation of reliable and objective detection systems, causal relation charts, and education/training. These factors taken together constitute a systems approach for solving the problem of preanalytic errors.

STANDARDS OF CARE

- The preanalytic phase of laboratory testing is manually intensive and prone to system flaws and operator error; a systems approach is required to avoid these kinds of errors.
- Failure to properly identify a patient, specimen, or test order can be considered a "misidentification" error and is actually a common preanalytic error in laboratory testing that can result in minor inconvenience (e.g., redrawing or relabeling) or in serious consequences (e.g., wrong patient or delay in diagnosis); the "paperwork" must be considered an integral and important part of patient care.
- Quality programs developed around the preanalytic phase of laboratory testing are required to avoid preanalytic errors; when errors occur, a root cause analysis must be done to identify any systems flaws that may contribute to such errors.

ANALYTIC ERRORS IN THE CLINICAL MICROBIOLOGY LABORATORY

In contrast to preanalytic errors in laboratory testing, analytic errors have been carefully addressed in both the clinical microbiology laboratory and in the laboratory as a whole. Bartlett et al. have comprehensively reviewed the process of managing quality in the clinical microbiology laboratory, and this review continues to serve as an ongoing template for a systems approach to quality. This does not mean that the analytic phase of testing in the clinical microbiology laboratory is error-free. Indeed, the detection and prevention of clinical microbiology laboratory–associated errors have been recognized and addressed by the American Society for Clinical Microbiology in their *Cumitech* series. The *Cumitech* series is designed to provide consensus recommendations regarding the judicious use of clinical microbiology and immunology laboratories; each series is written by a team of clinicians, laboratorians, and other knowledgeable stakeholders to provide a broad overview of various important aspects of infectious diseases testing. The discussion of analytic error that follows is based on the medical literature as well as the personal experience of the author and illustrates common medical errors that may occur in the clinical microbiology laboratory.

MISREADING OR MISINTERPRETATION OF GRAM STAIN OR OTHER STAINS

Misreading or misinterpretation of Gram stain or other stains is not a common problem in most clinical microbiology laboratories, but this error does occasionally happen. Technical issues usually contribute to this problem when it happens. These technical issues should be understood.

The well-recognized difficulty of diagnosing cryptococcal meningitis provides a useful example of cases where a misread Gram stain of the CSF may contribute to diagnostic confusion. The Gram stain of CSF is recognized as critical in the diagnostic evaluation of a patient with suspected meningitis, and positive Gram stains revealing microorganisms are used to direct initial therapy. Clinicians and laboratory personnel usually do not consider a false-positive Gram stain from CSF to be a potential problem. However, it must be appreciated that such false-positive Gram stains can occur.

In general, the microscopic examination of CSF in the diagnosis of meningitis is quite sensitive, ranging from 67% to 92%. It is rare for CSF examinations to incorrectly suggest the presence of microorganisms. *C. neoformans* is known to be confusing on Gram stain; both gram-positive and gram-negative misidentification is reported. A high index of suspicion for cryptococcal meningitis along with the use of the cryptococcal antigen test is a key factor in the diagnosis of such cases and will help avoid delays in treatment.

Clearly, the rapid and accurate detection and characterization of microorganisms encountered in purulent CSF from patients with meningitis are important. Quality assessment programs in the clinical microbiology laboratory include both internal and external proficiency testing as well as the testing of microbiology technologists for colorblindness. Such competency assessment in the clinical microbiology laboratory is an important, ongoing function that prevents such errors. In addition, most clinical microbiology laboratories routinely have a senior microbiologist review any positive Gram stains from CSF. Other causes of false-positive Gram stains from CSF are not infrequently described and do not include misreading the Gram stain. Instead, contamination with nonviable bacteria from various products used in the process is the cause of such false-positive Gram stains of CSF.

Factitious meningitis due to nonviable bacteria in commercial lumbar puncture trays was first reported in the mid-1970s and still occurs. The medical products industry has effectively ensured the sterility of commercial medical devices, but the procedures used to sterilize these products do not prevent the presence of nonviable microorganisms. Therefore, physicians and laboratory personnel must be aware that such false-positive Gram stains may occur. Although specimen tubes in lumbar puncture trays are the most common cause of factitious meningitis, other sources of nonviable microorganisms such as cytocentrifuge funnels and Gram-stain reagents may be a source. The laboratory must review any specimen showing microorganisms on direct smears that fail to grow. If factitious organisms are suspected, the physician should be notified. If possible, a repeat CSF specimen should be obtained using new, clean, and sterile glass tubes. Any cluster of such cases should be reported to the Food and Drug Administration (FDA).

Streptococcuss pneumoniae is a common cause of community-acquired meningitis in pediatric patients, but *Acinetobacter baumannii,* which is a short, plump, gram-negative rod that is difficult to destain, may also be misidentified as a gram-positive *Diplococcus.* Broad-spectrum antimicrobial therapy will provide coverage against this isolate. *A. baumannii* rarely causes community-acquired meningitis, although it has been reported as a cause of community-acquired pneumonia. When *A. baumannii* is seen as a cause of meningitis in a child, it usually follows a neurosurgical procedure and is multidrug resistant.

An issue with the Gram stain that is well known to microbiologists but not to physicians is Gram stain variability in select bacteria, including *Bacillus* species. *Bacillus* infections have been reported in orthopedic trauma cases. *Bacillus* species including *Bacillus cereus* are known to be gram-variable and can stain as gram-negative bacilli as well as gram-positive filamentous forms that show beading and can be confused with *Nocardia* species. *B. cereus* produces multiple beta-lactamases, which include a metallo-beta-lactamase. These beta-lactamases are very potent against beta-lactam agents, including the third-generation cephalosporins. Imipenem and other carbapenem agents seem to be active against *B. cereus* despite the presence of this metallo-beta-lactamase. However, carbapenem-resistant strains of *B. cereus* have been reported. Vancomycin or clindamycin are preferred choices for therapy of *B. cereus* infections.

Morphologic changes can sometimes be seen in gram-negative bacilli that are exposed to certain beta-lactam agents; for example, piperacillin interacting with penicillin-binding proteins may result in cell elongation without division. These filamentous forms may appear by Gram stain to be a fungal pathogen.

Prompt Gram staining of positive blood cultures is recognized as an important factor in directing antimicrobial therapy and has been shown to decrease mortality. As mentioned earlier, physicians rarely question the accuracy of such Gram stains. Yet, the exigencies of the staining properties of certain species of bacteria as well as human interpretive error can result in misinterpretation of a Gram stain from a positive blood culture. Indeed, misinterpretation of Gram stains from positive blood cultures has been reported for certain species of bacteria as well as for instances of under- or overdecolorization of the Gram stain. In one report, two systematic errors were noted. In 11 cases, *Bacillus* species were read as gram-negative bacilli (this is known to be a problem with this species), and in five cases, *Acinetobacter* species were read as gram-positive cocci or gram-positive bacilli (also a known problem with this species).

Underdecolorization and overdecolorization of the Gram stain are related to the use of acetone and isopropanol in the decolorization step. Acetone is too strong a decolorizer and isopropanol is too weak a decolorizer for gram-positive microorganisms. Therefore, most Gram stain kits use a mixture of one part acetone to three parts of isopropanol. The decolorization step should be done until the solvent running from the slide is colorless. Safranin or fuchsin is used as a counterstain and should be applied for 30 to 60 seconds. Prolonged application may cause gram-positive microorganisms to appear gram negative, while short application may cause gram-negative microorganisms to appear gram positive. The timing and the acetone/isopropanol ratio as well as the species of microorganism all are important factors in the Gram stain. For Gram stains of clinical specimens that include polymorphonuclear cells in the background, a good quality-control indicator is that occasionally the nucleus of a polymorphonuclear cell should stain purple. If most of the nuclei are staining purple, the stain is underdecolorized. If no purple nuclei can be seen after reviewing multiple fields, the stain is overdecolorized. If a Gram stain is considered under- or overdecolorized, the slide can be washed with xylene and the stain repeated.

Clearly, the answer to the question, "Can we always trust the Gram stain?" is "No." Misread Gram stains from positive blood cultures are generally recognized within one to two days when the microorganism grown on plates is recognized as being inconsistent with the Gram stain report; an amended report should be done. In addition, the physician should be notified by telephone.

Artifacts and organism mimickers can pose many problems in the diagnosis of infection. Of these problems, fungal elements from contamination during slide preparation are the most difficult to deal with because these will stain with Gomori methenamine silver (GMS) and periodic acid-Schiff (PAS) stains. Pathologists and microbiologists must assess the tissue inflammatory response when fungal elements are seen; if the cellular response is inconsistent, fungal contamination during slide preparation must be considered. An additional mimicker of fungal yeast elements can be seen in H&E stains from dermal lesions in which there is inflammation and plasma cells. This mimic is Russell bodies, which are intracytoplasmic immunoglobulin bodies in plasma cells. Russell bodies have been reported to cause confusion with blastomycosis as well as other pathogenic fungi such as *Histoplasma*, *Cryptococcus*, and *Candida* species that have yeast forms. Russell bodies are of variable size and lack the budding characteristics of these pathogenic fungi. Although Russell bodies are positive with PAS stains, they stain brown-gray with GMS, not black as would be expected.

The evaluation of frozen sections also poses certain problems with speciation. Even with special GMS or PAS stains, identifying a specific fungal microorganism from tissue may be difficult even for experienced pathologists and microbiologists. Morphologic identification can be a useful tool for the preliminary diagnosis of fungal infection, but culture remains the gold standard for speciation. All should be used concurrently to ensure that an accurate diagnosis is made. For example, lack of budding in a frozen section stain can make *Blastomyces dermatitidis* difficult to distinguish from Coccidioides. Moreover, empty, overlapping spherules in Coccidioides can mimic budding yeast and be mistaken for *B. dermatitidis* broad-based yeast in the process of budding. The Alcian blue or an acid-fast stain can be used to distinguish between Coccidioides and Blastomyces; Coccidioides is negative and Blastomyces is weakly positive. Some recommend identifying the presence of at least one intact spherule containing endospores before making a diagnosis of Coccidioides in tissue. Other special stains can be used to distinguish Blastomyces from Cryptococcus. Cryptococcus usually will stain strongly with mucicarmine; the occasional capsule-deficient forms of cryptococci stain with melanin. In contrast, the cell wall of Blastomyces is only weakly positive when stained with mucicarmine and negative with melanin.

STANDARDS OF CARE

■ Gram stains or other stains can be misread and/or misinterpreted due to a number of technical reasons; these reasons are understood by clinical microbiologists and pathologists, but may not be understood by physicians taking care of the patient.

▓ When misreading and/or misinterpreting a stain occurs and is recognized, a corrected report must be entered into the health record; moreover, the clinicians involved should be called and told of this error.

▓ A root cause analysis should be done for misreading and/or misinterpreting a stain in order to determine if there are any recurring systems issues that can be corrected.

▓ Because many errors caused by misreading and/or misinterpreting a stain cannot be completely avoided due to technical reasons, it is important that microbiologists/pathologists maintain clear communication channels with clinicians in order to quickly resolve and correct such errors when they occur.

MISIDENTIFICATION OF MICROORGANISM

Misidentification of a microorganism does not occur frequently, but can happen. Often there are technical issues that must be appreciated. Correction of the misidentification in the medical record and timely communication of the misidentification are important.

Automated identification systems are known for misidentification of isolates of the *Burkholderia cepacia* complex (BCC), and molecular methods for confirmatory identification of BCC are highly recommended, such as amplification and sequencing of a 500-bp fragment of the 16S rRNA gene.

Burkholderia pseudomallei is the cause of melioidosis, a serious infection common in Southwest Asia. Treatment of any infection caused by *B. pseudomallei* is difficult, and there is a high rate of relapse if prolonged therapy is not completed. Generally, two weeks of intravenous therapy with ceftazidime or a carbapenem is given followed by at least four months of oral sulfamethoxizole/trimethoprim. Such cases also raise issues regarding the safety of laboratory personnel exposed to the pathogen. Automated systems for identification and antimicrobial susceptibility testing of bacterial isolates, such as the BD Phoenix Automated Biology System, have become standard in most clinical laboratories. Identification of bacterial isolates is dependent on the database of the automated system; *B. pseudomallei* is not in the database of the Phoenix System. Currently, the most rapid and accurate identification method for *B. pseudomallei* is a manual method that uses the API 20NE system combined with a noncommercial latex agglutination test. Molecular methods are accurate, but they take more time. The limitations of automated systems must be understood by clinical microbiologists in order to avoid this type of identification error.

Other identification methods are known to have difficulty distinguishing *Streptococcus constellatus* and other members of the *Streptococcus anginosus* (also known as *Streptococcus milleri*) group from group C streptococci (*Streptococcus equisimilis*). Many clinical microbiology laboratories presumptively identify beta-hemolytic streptococci on the basis of Lancefield grouping. Some of the group C streptococcal bacteremia cases reported in the medical literature may actually represent bacteremia by members of the *S. anginosus* group. Differentiation of group C streptococci from members of the *S. anginosus* group is best accomplished by the Voges-Proskauer (VP) test; members of the *S. anginosus* group produce acetoin whereas *S. equisimilis* does not. The Phoenix Automated Microbiology System cannot be expected to detect diacetyl (caramel odor); moreover, the Phoenix Streptococcal Panel does not include the VP test.

Isolation of a member of the *S. anginosus* group from a blood culture is a "sentinel result," because these pathogens can be associated with abscesses and/or suppurative thrombophlebitis. It is important that clinical microbiologists appreciate and alert clinicians to the potential pathogenicity of *S. anginosus*. This type of sentinel result has been termed a "vital value"; alerting clinicians regarding such a result can promote patient safety by preventing a medical error and is an example of "enhanced clinical consulting."

Another issue arises with misidentification of *Mycobacterium abscessus*, which may result in a substantial delay in the administration of optimal antimicrobial therapy against this pathogen. *M. abscessus* is a member of the rapidly growing mycobacteria that are unusual causes of endocarditis. Rapidly growing mycobacteria can easily be misidentified as *Nocardia* spp. or *Corynebacterium* spp. In a European quality control report, *Mycobacterium fortuitum* specimens labeled as "pus from an abscess" were sent to 50 clinical microbiology laboratories for proficiency testing. Only 13 of the 50 laboratories correctly identified *M. fortuitum*. These specimens were misidentified as *Nocardia* spp. (23 laboratories) or *Corynebacterium* spp. (14 laboratories). Acid-fast staining of gram-positive bacilli should be routinely included in the identification procedure; if acid-fast staining results are positive, isolates should be sent to a reference laboratory for definitive identification as well as for susceptibility testing.

Conventional diagnosis of mycobacterial infection uses acid-fast staining, culture, and phenotypic characterization of culture isolates; cultures may require weeks or months before results are available. Accordingly, nucleic acid probe- and amplification-based molecular methods have been developed for identification of mycobacterial culture isolates as well as for direct detection of mycobacteria in clinical specimens. These molecular methods have greatly reduced the time to diagnosis of tuberculosis. However, molecular methods have their own set of problems, such as the potential for misidentification of a microorganism owing to a false-positive result from a molecular amplification test for tuberculosis. The Gen-Probe Amplified *Mycobacterium tuberculosis* Direct (MTD) test is a rapid molecular test that uses isothermal transcription-mediated amplification and a hybridization protection assay to detect nucleic acid from *M. tuberculosis* complex in clinical specimens including lymph nodes. False-positive results may lead to a misdiagnosis of tuberculosis and weeks of unnecessary antituberculous therapy. A high concentration of *Mycobacterium leprae* in a clinical specimen, for example, can lead to a false-positive result for tuberculosis with the Gen-Probe MTD test.

The Roche COBAS AMPLICOR system is a fully automated RNA and DNA amplification and detection system for routine diagnostic PCR. The menu of this system includes selected members of the *Mycobacterium* family, including *M. tuberculosis*, *M. avium*, and *Mycobacterium intracellulare*. Use of this system has also resulted in false-positives for *M. tuberculosis*.

The presence of *M. leprae* in clinical specimens tested by two different molecular assays can result in misidentification for other species of *Mycobacterium*. Clinical microbiologists should be aware of this potential for this type of misidentification of *M. leprae* using commercially available MTB molecular assays.

Another well-known problem with PCR testing in the clinical microbiology laboratory is PCR amplification carryover contamination and subsequent false-positive results. The procedure for the PCR assay for HSV-1 may be modified to include a repeat assay for any positive results. This will not prevent PCR amplification carryover contamination but will reduce the likelihood of a false-positive result being reported. Over the past two decades, PCR assays and other DNA/RNA amplification techniques have been utilized in clinical microbiology laboratories. Unfortunately, the exquisite sensitivity of these assays makes them vulnerable to contamination. Potential sources of contamination include large numbers of target microorganisms/virions in clinical specimens as well as repeated amplification of the same target sequence, leading to accumulation of amplification product in the laboratory environment. The accumulation of amplification product is a critical issue and, if uncontrolled, will lead to contamination of laboratory reagents, equipment, and even the ventilation system. Accordingly, clinical microbiology laboratories utilizing PCR for diagnostic purposes have established protocols to minimize this problem. Nevertheless, false-positive results from PCR amplification carryover contamination in molecular assays continue to occur occasionally despite the best efforts of a laboratory. When a false-positive result is recognized, a corrected report should be issued. In addition, a root cause analysis should be done to be sure that there is no recurring systems issue that can be corrected. Finally, communication with clinicians about amplification carryover contamination in a PCR assay is very important; many clinicians do not fully understand this issue and may attribute such false positives to technologist error.

STANDARDS OF CARE

- Misidentification of microorganisms can occur for a number of technical reasons; microbiologists are familiar with these technical reasons for misidentification, but clinicians may not understand these issues.
- When misidentification occurs and is recognized, a corrected report must be entered into the health record; moreover, the clinicians involved should be called and told of this error and why such errors occur despite best efforts to prevent them.
- A root cause analysis should be done for misidentification in order to determine if there are any recurring systems issues that can be corrected.
- Molecular methods such as PCR can assist in the correct identification of microorganisms, but may require additional time; moreover, PCR methods have their own set of problems with false-positive results due to PCR amplification carryover contamination being the most critical problem.
- Because some errors caused by misidentification cannot be avoided due to technical reasons,

it is important that microbiologists/pathologists maintain clear communication channels with clinicians in order to quickly explain and resolve such errors when they occur.

SUSCEPTIBILITY TESTING ERROR

Susceptibility testing error does not occur frequently in the clinical microbiology laboratory, but such errors can happen. Often there is a technical reason for such errors; automated susceptibility testing systems have been involved in such errors.

Most clinical microbiology laboratories today rely on automated systems such as the Phoenix Automated Microbiology System for identification and susceptibility testing. Such systems can give inaccurate results for selected antimicrobial agents and microorganism combinations; aminoglycoside resistance and susceptibility testing errors for *A. baumannii* is one of these combinations. It is recommended that confirmation by a manual method be done for this combination.

The performance of susceptibility testing in a clinical microbiology laboratory depends on robust methodology, good laboratory practices, and clearly delineated antimicrobial breakpoints. Moreover, routine susceptibility testing must be checked with both internal and external quality control programs. At one time, the results of susceptibility testing were so disconnected from actual clinical outcomes that one microbiologist was compelled to ask "*In vitro* Veritas?" Fortunately, this message was heard and improvements were implemented. Today, susceptibility testing has been greatly improved thanks to organizations such as the National Committee for Clinical Laboratory Standards (NCCLS), which has been renamed the Clinical Laboratory Standards Institute (CLSI). The published standards/guidelines from the NCCLS/CLSI provide the basis for uniform susceptibility testing procedures in the clinical microbiology laboratory.

Although there are still occasional errors, these errors should be recognized and quickly corrected.

Both clinicians and the clinical microbiology laboratory face uncertainty when the results of a susceptibility test are not consistent with the established susceptibility patterns for a particular species. The availability and reflex use of a confirmation test may be critical for directing proper antimicrobial therapy. For example, the CDC recommend that clinical microbiology laboratories perform a modified Hodge test or use PCR testing to confirm the presence of KPC carbapenemases in isolates with reduced susceptibility to carbapenems. Clinical microbiology laboratories must take an aggressive approach to detecting carbapenemases in order to provide clinicians with clinically relevant susceptibility results.

One of the critical functions of the director of a clinical microbiology laboratory is to select and monitor the susceptibility testing procedures and results so that these provide clinicians with relevant information. As resistance is constantly changing, the director must be aware of newly emerging resistance mechanisms and utilize new molecular technologies to detect such mechanisms.

STANDARDS OF CARE

- Susceptibility testing errors can occur for a number of technical reasons; microbiologists are familiar with these technical reasons for susceptibility testing errors, but clinicians may not understand these issues.
- When a susceptibility testing error occurs and is recognized, a corrected report must be entered into the health record; moreover, the clinicians involved should be called and told of this error.
- A root cause analysis should be done for susceptibility testing errors in order to determine if there are any recurring systems issues that can be corrected.

▓ Molecular methods such as PCR are being evaluated
in place of phenotypic susceptibility testing methods, but are not yet widely used; it should be anticipated that PCR methods also would have their own
set of problems.

▓ Because some errors caused by susceptibility testing cannot be avoided due to technical reasons, it is
important that microbiologists/pathologists maintain clear communication channels with clinicians in
order to quickly resolve such errors when they occur.

POSTANALYTIC ERRORS IN THE CLINICAL MICROBIOLOGY LABORATORY

The postanalytic phase in laboratory testing includes
the reporting of the laboratory result to the clinician
as well as the clinician's interpretation of that result.
Reporting of laboratory results has received a great
deal of attention since the early 1970s when the concept of *critical values* in laboratory medicine was first
introduced. This concept has been expanded to include
a "vital value." A vital value is defined as a laboratory
result that is just as important as a critical value, but
one for which timing is not as crucial. Many of the test
results from the clinical microbiology laboratory logi-
cally can be defined as vital values. Microbiology test
results that are of vital value require timely notification of the health care provider; most microbiology
laboratories call nurses or physicians for such results.

Notification of the health care provider for critical
values has become an established laboratory policy in
all medical centers. Indeed, physician communication
has become a focal point in efforts to promote patient
safety by preventing medical errors. Timely communication of important laboratory data has long been recognized as essential for providing optimal health care.

The responsibility for interpretation of laboratory
data has not been as clear as the reporting of these data.

The role of surgical pathology in the interpretation of histopathologic results has long been recognized. However, similar interpretation of laboratory data by the clinical pathologist has been less clear, and this concept is only recently coming to the forefront. The responsibilities of clinical pathologists, like the surgical pathologist, should extend into the postanalytic phase of the laboratory testing to assist clinicians in reviewing and understanding the results, and often providing an interpretation and/or recommending a future course of action. Failure to provide such information may result in a postanalytic error. The discussion of postanalytic error that follows is based on the medical literature as well as the personal experience of the author and includes common postanalytic medical errors from the perspective of the clinical microbiology laboratory.

FAILURE OF CLINICIANS TO CONSIDER AND/OR CORRECTLY INTERPRET MICROBIOLOGY RESULTS

Failure of clinicians to consider and/or to correctly interpret microbiology results is not a frequent cause of medical errors, but the problem does occur. Consultation with infectious disease clinicians and/or the clinical microbiology laboratory director can help avoid such errors.

The diagnosis of Lyme disease can be difficult; overdiagnosis and overtreatment of Lyme disease is a recognized problem. In one notable case, a patient died from a complication of her chronic indwelling central venous catheter, which had been placed for prolonged intravenous antimicrobial therapy for chronic Lyme disease. The diagnosis of chronic Lyme disease, however, was not fully documented. The chronic symptoms of this patient were nonspecific, and the results of her diagnostic evaluation for Lyme disease did not support this diagnosis. In this case, the diagnosis of Lyme disease was based on the result of one positive PCR assay out of a total of 11 PCR assays done on this patient; this finding may have been the result of PCR amplification carryover contamination. Another similar case with false-positive results for PCR testing for Lyme disease has been reported in the medical literature. Sequential testing with enzyme immunoassay antibody assay for *B. burgdorferi* and confirmation by Western blot is the most accurate method for ruling in or out the possibility of Lyme disease.

Diagnosis of Whipple's disease may pose similar difficulties, such as contradictory results between PAS staining of duodenal biopsies and PCR techniques. The problem of false-positive PCR results for Whipple's disease is also well known. Contradictory results warrant antimicrobial therapy with oral sulfamethoxazole/trimethoprim or oral tetracycline as this therapy can result in rapid improvement of the clinical status. Critical review of the diagnostic results, including meticulous re-evaluation of all specimens and repeated sampling, is warranted. Careful review of previous culture results is always advisable, as is telephone notification of this result to the clinicians caring for this patient.

In another case, a patient was preoperatively suspected of having a brain tumor based on imaging findings but was eventually diagnosed with a brain gumma based on brain histopathology and CSF analysis. However, this patient's medical history revealed that she had been engaged in prostitution in the past; a serum Venereal Disease Research Laboratory (VDRL) result was positive, as was a fluorescent treponemal antibody-absorption (FTA-ABS) IgG test. Based on this serologic information and the imaging studies of the brain, neurosyphilis and a brain gumma should have been considered. If neurosyphilis had been suspected, the diagnosis could have been made by analysis of the CSF; this analysis includes a CSF VDRL and FTA-ABS IgG test.

Related problems may arise in diagnosing acute HIV infection as this infection is characterized by a negative or weakly positive ELISA test for HIV, a negative or indeterminate Western blot analysis for HIV-1, and high-level viremia detected by nucleic acid testing. Quantitative testing for HIV-1 nucleic acids may be needed to make this diagnosis. The fact that an ELISA test for HIV is weakly positive and the Western blot analysis for HIV-1 is negative should not prevent the correct test from being done.

Acute HIV-1 infection is also a recognized cause of a mononucleosis-like syndrome and should be considered in the differential diagnosis for patients presenting with a classic mononucleosis-like triad of fever, sore throat, and lymphadenopathy. The diagnosis of acute HIV-1 largely depends on quantitative testing for HIV-1 nucleic acids. Finally, acute HIV-1 infection presenting as a mononucleosis-like syndrome also must be considered in adolescents as up to half of all new HIV-1 infections occur in this age group.

Diagnosing even a relatively common infectious disease such as mononucleosis may be difficult when the clinical presentation is not what is usually seen.

A final case illustrating incorrect interpretation of microbiology results involves lack of recognition of *Staphylococcus lugdunensis* as a pathogen. *S. lugdunensis* is a member of the coagulase-negative staphylococci and, as such, may not be considered a pathogen. However, *S. lugdunensis* has become recognized as an atypically virulent pathogen with a unique clinical profile. For instance, although coagulase-negative staphylococci are rarely found in a breast abscess, such infections do occur. Serious consequences may occur if an *S. lugdunensis* isolate is in endocarditis. Although rare, *S. lugdunensis* is now a recognized cause of endocarditis and can cause destructive native valve endocarditis. Because *S. lugdunensis* isolated from blood cultures in children or adults may indicate infectious endocarditis, coagulase-negative staphylococci from blood cultures should be speciated.

STANDARDS OF CARE

▨ Failure of clinicians to consider and/or correctly interpret microbiology results is less likely in an age of electronic information when the medical literature is available on one's telephone; given this fact, this type of error is less forgivable.

▨ When clinicians do fail to consider and/or correctly interpret microbiology results, it is likely to be an oversight; attention to detail is important when considering the volume of information generated by a medical evaluation.

▨ Newer molecular tests and/or newer antigen tests are perhaps easier to misinterpret, in part, because of their newness; their sensitivity and specificity may still be evolving.

▨ Recognition of the pathogenesis and virulence of microorganisms are constantly evolving; do not assume that a microorganism is not a pathogen simply because it was not recognized as such in the past.

BIBLIOGRAPHY

Adam O, Auperin A, Wilquin F, et al. Treatment with piperacillin-tazobactam and false-positive *Aspergillus* galactomannan antigen test results for patients with hematological malignancies. *Clin Infect Dis.* 2004;38:917–920.

Aggarwal M, Rein J. Acute human immunodeficiency virus syndrome in an adolescent. *Pediatrics.* 2003;112:e323.

Aguero-Rosenfeld ME. Lyme disease: laboratory issues. *Infect Dis Clin N Am.* 2008;22:301–313.

Aguero-Rosenfeld ME, Wang G, Schwartz I, Wormser GP. Diagnosis of Lyme borreliosis. *Clin Microbiol Rev.* 2005;18:484–509.

Ahmed A, Engelberts MF, Boer KR, et al. Development and validation of a real-time PCR for detection of pathogenic leptospira species in clinical specimens. *PLoS ONE.* 2009;4:e7093.

Akers KS, Chaney C, Barsoumian A, et al. Aminoglycoside resistance and susceptibility testing errors in *Acinetobacter baumannii-calcoaceticus* complex. *J Clin Microbiol*. 2010;48:1132–1138.

Akhan SE, Dogan Y, Akhan S, et al. Pelvic actinomycosis mimicking ovarian malignancy: three cases. *Eur J Gynaecol Oncol*. 2008;29:294–297.

Al Dalhouk S, Tomaso H, Nockler K, et al. Laboratory-based diagnosis of brucellosis—a review of the literature. Part I: techniques for direct detection and identification of *Brucella* spp. *Clin Lab*. 2003;49:487–505.

Al Dalhouk S, Tomaso H, Nockler K, et al. Laboratory-based diagnosis of brucellosis—a review of the literature. Part II: serological tests for brucellosis. *Clin Lab*. 2003;49:577–589.

Al-Eissa Y, Al-Zamil F, Al-Mugeiren M, et al. Childhood brucellosis: a deceptive infectious disease. *Scand J Infect Dis*. 1991;23:129–133.

Alleva M, Guida RA, Romo T III, Kimmelman CP. Mycobacterial cervical lymphadenitis: a persistent diagnostic problem. *Laryngoscope*. 1988;98:855–857.

Amarzooqi S, Leber A, Kahwash S. Artifacts and organism mimickers in pathology. Case examples and review of the literature. *Adv Anat Pathol*. 2010;17:277–281.

Amornchai P, Chierakul W, Wuthieckanum V, et al. Accuracy of *Burkholderia pseudomallei* identification using the API 20NE system and a latex agglutination test. *J Clin Microbiol*. 2007;45:3774–3776.

Amsterdam D, Barenfanger J, Campos J, et al. *Cumitech 41. Detection and Prevention of Clinical Microbiology Laboratory-Associated Errors*. James W. Snyder, coordinating ed. Washington, DC: ASM Press; 2004:1–14.

Anastasi J, Ashwood E, Baron B, et al. The clinical pathologist as consultant. *Am J Clin Pathol*. 2011;135:11–12.

Antopolski M, Hiller N, Salameh S, et al. Splenic infarction: 10 years of experience. *Am J Emerg Med*. 2009;27:262–265.

Araj GF. Human brucellosis: a classical infectious disease with persistent diagnostic challenges. *Clin Lab Sci*. 1999;12:207–212.

Araj GF. Update on laboratory diagnosis of human brucellosis. *Int J Antimicrob Agents*. 2010;36(suppl 1):S12–S17.

Ashford RU, Scolyer PA, McCarthy SW, et al. The role of intra-operative pathological evaluation in the management of musculoskeletal tumors. *Recent Results Cancer Res.* 2009;179:11–24.

Aslanzadeh J. Preventing PCR amplification carryover contamination in a clinical laboratory. *Ann Clin Lab Sci.* 2004;34:389–396.

Asnis DS, St John S, Tickoo R, Arora A. *Staphylococcus lugdunensis* breast abscess: is it real? *Clin Infect Dis.* 2003;36:1348.

Atay Y, Altintas A, Tuncer I, Cennet A. Ovarian actinomycosis mimicking malignancy. *Eur J Gynaecol Oncol.* 2005;26:663–664.

Atge JP. *Aspergillus fumigatus* and aspergillosis. *Clin Microbiol Rev.* 1999;12:310–350.

Azuma I, Kaanetsuna F, Tanaka Y, et al. Chemical and immunological properties of galactomannans obtained from *Histoplasma duboisii*, *Histoplasma capsulatum*, *Paracoccidioides brasiliensis*, and *Blastomyces dermatitidis*. *Mycopathol Mycol Appl.* 1974;54:111–125.

Babayigit A, Olimez D, Sozmen SC, et al. Infection caused by *Nocardia farcinica* mimicking pulmonary metastasis in an adolescent girl. *Pediatr Emerg Care.* 2010;26:203–205.

Baebler JW, Kleiman MB, Cohen M, et al. Differentiation of lymphoma from histoplasmosis in children with mediastinal masses. *J Pediatr.* 1984;104:706–709.

Bain BJ. Russell bodies. *Am J Hematol.* 2009;84:439.

Bajani MD, Ashvord DA, Bragg SL, et al. Evaluation of four commercially available rapid serologic test for diagnosis of leptospirosis. *J Clin Microbiol.* 2003;41:802–809.

Balasingham SV, Davidsen T, Szpinda I, et al. Molecular diagnostics in tuberculosis: basis and implications for therapy. *Mol Diagn Ther.* 2009;13:137–151.

Barbour AG. Laboratory aspects of Lyme borreliosis. *Clin Microbiol Rev.* 1988;1:399–414.

Barenfanger J, Graham DR, Kolluri L, et al. Decreased mortality associated with prompt Gram staining of blood cultures. *Am J Clin Pathol.* 2008;130:870–876.

Barnes PJ. Anti-inflammatory actions of glucocorticoids: molecular mechanisms. *Clin Sci.* 1998;94:557–572.

Bartlett JG. Diagnostic test for etiologic agents of community-acquired pneumonia. *Infect Dis Clin North Am.* 2004;18:809–827.

Bartlett RC, Mazens-Sullivan M, Tetreault JZ, et al. Evolving approaches to management of quality in clinical microbiology. *Clin Microbiol Rev.* 1994;7:55–88.

Bazemore AW, Smucker DR. Lymphadenopathy and malignancy. *Am Fam Physician.* 2002;66:2103–2110.

Belko J, Goldmann DA, Macone A, Zaidi AKM. Clinically significant infections with organisms of the *Streptococcus milleri* group. *Pediatr Infect Dis.* 2002;21:715–726.

Bell CA, Patel R. A real-time combined polymerase chain reaction assay for the rapid detection and differentiation of *Anaplasma phagocytophilum, Ehrlichia chaffeensis,* and *Ehrlichia ewingii. Diagn Microbiol Infect Dis.* 2005;53:301–306.

Bell SK, Rosenberg ES. Case records of the Massachusetts General Hospital. Case 11-2009: a 47-year-old man with fever, headache, rash, and vomiting. *N Engl J Med.* 2009;360:1540–1548.

Benevento G, Avellini C, Terrosu G, et al. Diagnosis and assessment of Crohn's disease: the present and the future. *Expert Rev Gastroenterol Hepatol.* 2010;4:757–766.

Benjamin DR. Clinical pathologist. A physician's consultant. *Arch Pathol Lab Med.* 1984;108:782.

Berlin L, Pincus JH. Cryptcoccal meningitis. False-negative antigen test results and cultures in nonimmunosuppressed patients. *Arch Neurol.* 1989;46:1312–1316.

Bert F, Bariou-Lancelin M, Lambert-Zechovsky N. Clinical significance of bacteremia involving the *"Streptococcus milleri"* group: 51 cases and review. *Clin Infect Dis.* 1998;27:385–387.

Beveridge TJ. Mechanism of Gram variability in select bacteria. *J Bacteriol.* 1990;172:1609–1620.

Bharti AR, Nally JE, Ricaldi JN, et al. Leptospirosis: a zoonotic disease of global importance. *Lancet Infect Dis.* 2003;3:757–771.

Bjorksten B, Boquist L. Histopathological aspects of chronic recurrent multifocal osteomyelitis. *J Bone Joint Surg Br.* 1980;62:376–380.

Bodmer T, Gurtner A, Scholkmann M, Matter L. Evaluation of the COBAS AMPLICOR MTB system. *J Clin Microbiol.* 1997;35:1604–1605.

Boggild AK, Page AV, Keystone JS, et al. Delay in diagnosis: malaria in a returning traveler. *CMAJ.* 2009; 180:1129–1131.

Borst A, Box ATA, Fluit AC. False-positive results and contamination in nucleic acid amplification assays: suggestions for a prevent and destroy strategy. *Eur J Clin Microbiol Infect Dis.* 2004;23:289–299.

Bottieau E, Clerinx J, Van den Enden E, et al. Fever after a stay in the tropics: diagnostic predictors of the leading tropical conditions. *Medicine.* 2007;86:18–25.

Bottone EJ. *Cryptococcus neoformans*: pitfalls in diagnosis through evaluation of Gram-stained smears of purulent exudates. *J Clin Microbiol.* 1980;12:790–791.

Bottone EJ. *Bacillus cereus*, a volatile human pathogen. *Clin Microbiol Rev.* 2010;23:382–398.

Bradley SF, Gordon JJ, Baumgartner DD, et al. Group C streptococcal bacteremia: analysis of 88 cases. *Rev Infect Dis.* 1991;13:270–280.

Branson D. Problems and errors in the clinical microbiology laboratory. *Am J Med Technol.* 1966;32:349–357.

Brigante G, Luzzaro F, Bettaccini A, et al. Use of the Phoenix Automated System for identification of *Streptococcus* and *Enterococcus* spp. *J Clin Microbiol.* 2006;44:3263–3267.

Brightbill TC, Ihmeidan IH, Post MJD, et al. Neurosyphilis in HIV-positive and HIV-negative patients: neuroimaging findings. *Am J Neuroradiol.* 1995;16:703–711.

Brisse S, Stefani S, Verhoef J, et al. Comparison evaluation of the BD Phoenix and VITEK 2 automated instruments for identification of isolated of the *Burkholderia cepacia* complex. *J Clin Microbiol.* 2002;40:1743–1748.

British Thoracic Society Standards of Care Committee. BTS guidelines for the management of community-acquired pneumonia in childhood. *Thorax.* 2002;57 (suppl 1):1–24.

Brogan O, Malone J, Fox C, Whyte AS. Lancefield grouping and smell of caramel for presumptive identification and assessment of pathogenicity in the *Streptococcus milleri* group. *J Clin Pathol.* 1997;50:332–335.

Brown JR, Skarin AT. Clinical mimics of lymphoma. *Oncologist.* 2004;9:406–416.

Brown-Elliott BA, Brown JM, Conville PS, Wallace RA Jr. Clinical and laboratory features of the *Nocardia* spp. based on current molecular taxonomy. *Clin Micro Rev.* 2006;19:259–282.

Bruck E. National Committee for Clinical Laboratory Standards. *Pediatrics.* 1980;65:187–188.

Brucker DA, Garcia LS, Shimizu RY, et al. Babesiosis: problems in diagnosis using autoanalyzers. *Am J Clin Pathol.* 1985;83:520–521.

Bucher C, von Graevenitz A. Differentiation in throat cultures of group C and G streptococci and *Streptococcus milleri* with identical antigens. *Eur J Clin Microbiol.* 1984:3:44–45.

Buckley JD, Joyce B, Garcia AJ, et al. Linking residency training effectiveness to clinical outcomes: a quality improvement approach. *Jt Comm J Qual Patient Saf.* 2010;36:203–208.

Bui MM, Smith P, Agresta SV, et al. Practical issues of intraoperative frozen section diagnosis of bone and soft tissue lesions. *Cancer Control.* 2008;15:7–12.

Burgert SJ, LaRocco MT, Wilansky S. Destructive native valve endocarditis caused by *Staphylococcus lugdunensis. South Med J.* 1999;92:812–814.

Bush MP, Kleinman SH, Tobler LH, et al. Virus and antibody dynamics in acute West Nile virus infection. *J Infect Dis.* 2008;198:984–993.

Calisher CH. Medically important arboviruses of the United States and Canada. *Clin Microbiol Rev.* 1994;7:89–116.

Caraway NP, Fanning CV, Stewart JM, et al. Coccidioidomycosis osteomyelitis masquerading as a bone tumor. A report of 2 cases. *Acta Cytol.* 2003;47:777–782.

Carlos FP, Menry MB. Psoas muscle abscess caused by *Mycobacterium tuberulosis* and *Staphylococcus aureus*: case report and review. *Am J Med Sci.* 2001;321:415–417.

Carr JM, Emery S, Stone BF, Tulin L. Babesiosis. Diagnostic pitfalls. *Am J Clin Pathol.* 1991;95:774–777.

Case records of the Massachusetts General Hospital. Weekly clinicopathological exercises. Case 35-1971. *N Engl J Med.* 1971;285:567–575.

Centers for Disease Control and Prevention. Case definitions for infectious conditions under public health surveillance. *MMWR Morb Mortal Wkly Rep.* 1997;46:12–13.

Centers for Disease Control and Prevention. *Brucella suis* infections associated with feral swine hunting—three states, 2007–2008. *MMWR Morb Mortal Wkly Rep.* 2009;58:618–621.

Centers for Disease Control and Prevention. *Final 2009 West Nile Virus Activity in the United States.* Atlanta, GA: Centers

for Disease Control and Prevention; 2009. http://www
.cdc.gov/ncidod/dvbid/westnile/surv&controlCase
Count09_detailed.htm. Accessed October 4, 2010.

Centers for Disease Control and Prevention. *Updated
Interim Recommendations for the Clinical Use of Antiviral
Medications in the Treatment and Prevention of Influenza for
the 2009–2010 Season.* Atlanta, GA: Centers for Disease
Control and Prevention; 2009.

Centor RM. Expand the pharyngitis paradigm for adolescents
and young adults. *Ann Intern Med.* 2009;151:812–815.

Chandor SB, Stemmer EA, Calvin JW, Connolly JE.
Mediastinal biopsy for indeterminate chest lesions.
Thorax. 1966;21:533–537.

Chang HC, Verhoeven W, Chay VM. Rubber foreign bodies in
puncture wounds of the foot in patients wearing rubber-
soled shoes. *Foot Ankle Int.* 2001;22:409–414.

Chang MJ, Barton LL. *Mycobacterium fortuitum* osteomyelitis of the calcaneus secondary to a puncture wound.
J Pediatr. 1974;85:517–519.

Chatwani A, Amin-Hanjani S. Incidence of actinomycosis associated with intrauterine devices. *J Reprod Med.*
1994;39:585–587.

Chedore P, Broukhanski G, Shainhouse Z, Jamieson F. False-
positive Amplified *Mycobacterium tuberculosis* Direct
Test results for samples containing *Mycobacterium leprae.*
J Clin Microbiol. 2006;44:612–613.

Chen MZ, Hsueh PR, Lee LN, et al. Severe community-
acquired pneumonia due to *Acinetobacter baumannii.*
Chest. 2001;120:1072–1077.

Cheng AC, Currie BJ. Melioidosis: epidemiology, pathophysiology, and management. *Clin Microbiol Rev.*
2005;18:383–416.

Cheng VC, Yew WW, Yuen KY. Molecular diagnostics in tuberculosis. *Eur J Clin Microbiol Infect Dis.*
2005;11:711–720.

Chew TA, Smith JM. Detection of diacetyl (caramel odor) in
presumptive identification of the *"Streptococcus milleri"*
group. *J Clin Microbiol.* 1992;30:3028–3029.

Chirinos JA, Lichstein DM, Garcia J, Tamariz LJ. The evolution
of Lemierre syndrome: report of 2 cases and review of
the literature. *Medicine (Baltimore).* 2002;81:458–465.

Chisholm CD, Schlesser JF. Plantar puncture wounds: controversies and treatment recommendations. *Ann Emerg Med.* 1989;18:1352–1357.

Christensen JB, Koeppe J. *Mycobacterium avium* complex cervical lymphadentitis in an immunocompetent adult. *Clin Vaccine Immunol.* 2010;17:1488–1490.

Chua CL. The value of cervical lymph node biopsy—a surgical audit. *Aust NZ J Surg.* 1986;56:335–339.

Clark RB. Imipenem resistance among *Acinetobacter baumannii*: association with reduced expression of a 33–36 kDa outer membrane protein. *J Antimicrob Chemother.* 1996;38:245–251.

Clinical and Laboratory Standards Institute. *Performance Standards for Antimicrobial Susceptibility Testing. Twentieth Informational Supplement. CLSI Document M100-S20-U.* Wayne, PA: Clinical and Laboratory Standards Institute; 2010.

Cochran AJ. Melanoma metastases through the lymphatic system. *Surg Clin North Am.* 2000;80:1683–1693.

Coffin CM, Spilker K, Zhou H, et al. Frozen section diagnosis in pediatric surgical pathology: a decade's experience in a children's hospital. *Arch Pathol Lab Med.* 2005;129:1619–1625.

Colby TV, Weiss RL. Current concepts of the surgical pathology of pulmonary infections. *Am J Surg Pathol.* 1987;11(suppl 1):S25–S37.

Colmenero JD, Morata P, Ruiz-Mesa JD, et al. Multiplex real-time polymerase chain reaction: a practical approach for rapid diagnosis of tuberculosis and brucellar vertebral osteomyelitis. *Spine.* 2010;35:E1392–E1396.

Correa AG, Starke JR. Nontuberculous mycobacterial disease in children. *Seminar Respir Infect.* 1996;11:262–271.

Cowgill R, Quan SH. Colonic actinomycosis mimicking carcinoma. *Dis Colon Rectum.* 1979;22:45–46.

Cragun WC, Barlett BL, Ellis MW, et al. The expanding spectrum of escar-associated rickettsioses in the United States. *Arch Dermatol.* 2010;146:641–648.

Cruz AT, Starke JR. Pediatric tuberculosis. *Pediatr Rev.* 2010;1:13–25.

Culafic DM, Lekic NS, Kerkez MD, Mijac DD. Liver actinomycosis mimicking liver tumour. *Vojnosanit Pregl.* 2009;66:924–927.

Currie BP, Freundlich LF, Soto MA, Casadevall A. False-negative cerebrospinal fluid cryptococcal latex agglutination test for patients with culture-positive cryptococcal meningitis. *J Clin Microbiol.* 1993;31:2519–2522.

D'Acremont V, Landry P, Mueller I, et al. Clinical and laboratory predictors of imported malaria in an outpatient setting: an aid to medical decision making in returning travelers with fever. *Am J Trop Med Hyg.* 2002;66:481–486.

Daily JP, Waldron MA. Case 22-2003: a 22-year-old man with chills and fever after a stay in South America. *N Engl J Med.* 2003;349:287–295.

Dandache P, Nadelman RB. Erythema migrans. *Infect Dis Clin N Am.* 2008;22:235–260.

De Champs C, Le Seaux S, Dubost JJ, et al. Isolation of *Pantoea agglomerans* in two cases of septic monoarthritis after plant thorn and wood sliver injuries. *J Clin Microbiol.* 2000;38:460–461.

De Groote MA, Huitt G. Infections due to rapidly growing mycobacteria. *Clin Infect Dis.* 2006;41:1756–1763.

DeForges L, Legrand P, Tankovic J, et al. Case of false-positive results of the urine antigen test for *Legionella pneumophila*. *Clin Infect Dis.* 1999;29:953–954.

Dexler JF, Helmer A, Kirberg H, et al. Poor clinical sensitivity of rapid antigen testing for influenza A pandemic (H1N1) 2009 virus. *Emerg Infect Dis.* 2009;15:1662–1664.

DiDomenico N, Link H, Knobel R, et al. COBAS AM. LICOR: fully automated RNA and DNA amplification and detection system for routine diagnostic PCR. *Clin Chem.* 1996;42:1915–1923.

Dieckman KP, Henke RP, Ovenbeck R. Renal actinomycosis mimicking renal carcinoma. *Eur Urol.* 2001;39:357–359.

Dighe AS, Rao A, Coakley AB, Lewandrowski KB. Analysis of laboratory critical values reporting in a large academic medical center. *Am J Clin Path.* 2006;125:758–764.

Doherty JF, Grant AD, Brycesson AD. Fever as the presenting complaint of travelers returning from the tropics. *QJM.* 1995;88:277–281.

Doig GS, Simpson F. Efficient literature searching: a core skill for the practice of evidence-base medicine. *Intensive Care Med.* 2003;29:2119–2127.

Donato AA, Chaudhary A. A 78-year-old man with the "summer flu" and cytopenias. *Clin Infect Dis*. 2009;48:1433, 1479–1480.

Dowell SF, Smith T, Leversedge K, Snitzer J. Failure of treatment of pneumonia associated with highly resistant pneumococci in a child. *Clin Infect Dis*. 1999;29:462–463.

Drobniewski FA. *Bacillus cereus* and related species. *Clin Microbiol Rev*. 1993;6:324–338.

Dubouix A, Bonnet E, Alvarez M, et al. *Bacillus cereus* infections in Traumatology-Orthopaedics Department: retrospective investigation and improvement of healthcare practices. *J Infection*. 2005;50:22–30.

Dumler JS, Madigan JE, Pusteria N, Bakken JS. Ehrlichioses in humans: epidemiology, clinical presentation, diagnosis, and treatment. *Clin Infect Dis*. 2007;45(suppl):S45–S51.

Dumler JS, Walker DH. Rocky Mountain spotted fever— changing ecology and persisting virulence. *N Engl J Med*. 2005;353:551–553.

Dunbar SA, Eason RA, Musher DM, Clarridge JE III. Microscopic examination and broth culture of cerebrospinal fluid in diagnosis of meningitis. *J Clin Microbiol*. 1998;36:1617–1620.

Duncan CJ, Gallacher K, Kennedy DH, et al. Infectious disease telephone consultations: numerous, varied, and an important educational resource. *J Infect*. 2007;54:515–516.

Durand DV, Lecomte C, Cathebras P, et al. Whipple disease. Clinical review of 52 cases. *Medicine*. 1997;76:170–184.

Durkin M, Witt J, LeMonte A, et al. Antigen assay with the potential to aid in diagnosis of blastomycosis. *J Clin Microbiol*. 2004;42:4873–4875.

Dykers TI, Brown KL, Gundersen CB, Beaty BJ. Rapid diagnosis of LaCrosse encephalitis: detection of specific immunoglobulin M in cerebrospinal fluid. *J Clin Microbiol*. 1985;22:740–744.

Dzirto L, Hubner M, Muller C, et al. A mimic of sarcoidosis. *Lancet*. 2007;369:1832.

Easton A. Leptospirosis in Philippine floods. *BMJ*. 1999; 319:212.

Ebbert JO, Dupras DM, Egwin PJ. Searching the medical literature using PubMed: a tutorial. *Mayo Clin Proc*. 2003;78:87–91.

Ecevit IZ, Clancy CJ, Schmalfuss IM, Nguyen MH. The poor prognosis of central nervous system cryptococcosis among nonimmunosuppressed patients: a call for better disease recognition and evaluation of adjuncts to antifungal therapy. *Clin Infect Dis.* 2006;42:1443–1447.

Efrati O, Sadeh-Gornik U, Modan-Moses D, et al. Flexible bronchoscopy and bronchoalveolar lavage in pediatric patients with lung disease. *Pediatr Crit Care Med.* 2009;10:80–84.

Egberts F, Moller M, Proksch E, Schwarz T. Multiple erythema migrans—manifestation of systemic cutaneous borreliosis. *J Dtsch Dermatol Ges.* 2008;6:350–353.

Ehrbar HU, Bauerfeind P, Dutly F, et al. PCR-positive tests for *Tropheryma whipplei* in patients without Whipple's disease. *Lancet.* 1999;353:2214.

Eilers RJ. Total quality control for the medical laboratory. *South Med J.* 1969;62:1362–1365.

Eremeea ME, Dasch GA, Silverman DJ. Evaluation of a PCR assay for quantification of *Rickettsia rickettsii* and closely related spotted fever group rickettsiae. *J Clin Microbiol.* 2003;41:5466–5472.

Ergul Z, Hoca O, Karahan MA, et al. A transverse colonic mass secondary to *Actinomyces* infection mimicking cancer. *Turk J Gastroenterol.* 2008;19:200–201.

Ericsson CD, Carmichael M, Pickering LK, et al. Erroneous diagnosis of meningitis due to false-positive Gram stains. *South Med J.* 1978;71:1524–1525.

Eshoo MW, Crowder CD, Li H, et al. Detection and identification of *Ehrlichia* species in blood by use of PCR and electrospray ionization mass spectrometry. *J Clin Microbiol.* 2010;48:472–478.

Evans DTP. *Actinomyces israelii* in the female genital tract: a review. *Genitourin Med.* 1993;69:54–59.

Ewig S, Schlochtermeier M, Goke N, Niederman MS. Applying sputum as a diagnostic tool in pneumonia. Limited yield, minimal impact on treatment decisions. *Chest.* 2002;121:1486–1492.

Fargen KM. Cerebral syphilitic gummata: a case presentation and analysis of 156 reported cases. *Neurosurgery.* 2009;64:568–575.

Feder HM, Whitaker DL. Misdiagnosis of erythema migrans. *Am J Med.* 1995;99:412–419.

Feigin RD, Lobes LA, Anderson D, Pickering L. Human leptospirosis from immunized dogs. *Ann Intern Med.* 1973;79:777–785.

Fenoliar F, Ampoux B, Raoult D. A paradoxical *Tropheryma whipplei* Western blot differentiates patients with Whipple disease from asymptomatic carriers. *Clin Infect Dis.* 2009;49:717–723.

Fenollar F, Fournier PE, Robert C, Raoult D. Use of genome selected repeated sequences increases the sensitivity of PCR detection of *Tropheryma whipplei. J Clin Microbiol.* 2004;42:401–103.

Fenollar F, Laouira S, Lepidi H, et al. Value of *Tropheryma whipplei* quantitative polymerase chain reaction assay for the diagnosis of Whipple disease: usefulness of saliva and stool specimens for first-line screening. *Clin Infect Dis.* 2008;47:659–667.

Fenollar F, Puechal X, Raoult D. Whipple's disease. *N Engl J Med.* 2007;356:55–66.

Fibin MR, Mylonakis EE, Callegari L, Legome E. Babesiosis. *J Emerg Med.* 2001;20:21–24.

Fiorino AS. Intrauterine contraceptive device–associated actinomycotic abscess and *Actinomyces* detection on cervical smear. *Obstet Gynecol.* 1996;87:142–149.

Fleming JL, Wiesner RH, Shorter RG. Whipple's disease: clinical, biochemical, and histopathologic features and assessment of treatment in 29 patients. *Mayo Clin Proc.* 1988;63:539–551.

Franco MP, Mulder M, Gilman RH, Smits HL. Human brucellosis. *Lancet Infect Dis.* 2007;7:775–786.

Frank KL, Del Pozo JL, Patel R. From clinical microbiology to infection pathogenesis: how daring to be different works for *Staphylococcus lugdunensis. Clin Microbiol Rev.* 2008;21:111–133.

Futterman D, Chabon B, Hoffman ND. HIV and AIDS in adolescents. *Pediatr Clin North Am.* 2000;47:171–188.

Gan HT, Chen YQ, Ouyang Q, et al. Differentiation between intestinal tuberculosis and Crohn's disease in endoscopic biopsy specimens by polymerase chain reaction. *Am J Gastroenterol.* 2002;97:1446–1451.

Garcia LS, Shimizu RY, Bruckner DA. Blood parasites: problems in diagnosis using automated differential instruments. *Diagn Microbiol Infect Dis.* 1986;4:173–176.

Garg P, Athmanathan S, Rao GM. *Mycobacterium chelonae* masquerading as *Corynebacterium* in a case of infectious keratitis: a diagnostic dilemma. *Cornea*. 1998;17:230–232.

Gayle A, Ringdahi E. Tick-borne diseases. *Am Fam Physician*. 2001;64:461–466.

Genta RM. Dysregulation of strongyloidiasis: a new hypothesis. *Clin Microbiol Rev*. 1992;5:345–355.

Gerhardt T, Wolff M, Fischer HP, et al. Pitfalls in the diagnosis of intestinal tuberculosis: a case report. *Scand J Gastroenterol*. 2005;40:240–243.

Gillies MJ, Farrugia M-K, Lakhoo K. An unusual case of a superior mediastinal mass in an infant. *Pediatr Surg Int*. 2008;24:485–486.

Ginsburg CM. An unusual cause of cervical lymphadenitis. *Laryngoscope*. 1977;87:1180–1181.

Gosselink C, Thomas J, Brahmbhatt S, et al. Nocardiosis causing pedal actinomycetoma: a case report and review of the literature. *J Foot Ankle Surg*. 2008;47:457–462.

Grace C, Alston WK, Ramundo M, et al. The complexity, relative value, and financial worth of curbside consultations in an academic infectious diseases unit. *Clin Infect Dis*. 2010;51:651–655.

Greenwood D. *In vitro* Veritas? Antimicrobial susceptibility tests and their clinical relevance. *J Infect Dis*. 1981;144:380–385.

Greer DM, Schaefer PW, Plotkin SR, et al. Case 11-2007: a 59-year-old man with neck pain, weakness in the arms, and cranial-nerve palsies. *N Engl J Med*. 2007;356:1561–1570.

Grosfeld JL, Skinner MA, Rescorla FJ, et al. Mediastinal tumors in children: experience with 196 cases. *Ann Surg Oncol*. 1994;1:121–127.

Grossman M, Shiramizu B. Evaluation of lymphadenopathy in children. *Curr Opin Pediatr*. 1994;1:68–76.

Habermann TM, Steensma DP. Lymphadenopathy. *Mayo Clin Proc*. 2000;75:723–732.

Haensch R, Seeliger H. Problems of differential diagnosis of blastomyces and Russell bodies. *Arch Dermatol Res*. 1981;270:381–385.

Hagelskjaer Kristensen L, Prag J. Human necrobacillosis, with emphasis on Lemierre's syndrome. *Clin Infect Dis*. 2000;31:524–532.

Han JK, Kerschner JE. *Streptococcus milleri*: an organism for head and neck infections and abscess. *Arch Otolaryngol Head Neck Surg*. 2001;127:650–654.

Hansmann Y, DeMartino S, Piemont Y, et al. Diagnosis of cat scratch disease with detection of *Bartonella henselae* by PCR: a study of patients with lymph node enlargement. *J Clin Microbiol*. 2005;43:3800–3806.

Harley WB, Blazer MB. Disseminated coccidioidomycosis associated with extreme eosinophilia. *Clin Infect Dis*. 1994;18:627–629.

Harper SA, Bradley JS, Englund JA, et al. Seasonal influenza in adults and children—diagnosis, treatment, chemo-prophylaxis, and institutional outbreak management: clinical practice guidelines of the Infectious Diseases Society of America. *Clin Infect Dis*. 2009;48:1003–1032.

Healy DP, Gardner JC, Puthoff BK, et al. Antibiotic-mediated bacterial filamentation: a potentially important laboratory phenomenon. *Clin Microbiol Newsl*. 2007;29:22–24.

Heelan JS, Corpus L, Kessimian N. False-positive reaction in the latex agglutination test for *Cryptococcus neoformans* antigen. *J Clin Microbiol*. 1991;29:1260–1261.

Heller HM, Telford SR III, Branda JA. Case records of the Massachusetts General Hospital. Case 10-2005. A 73-year-old man with weakness and pain in the legs. *N Engl J Med*. 2005;352:1358–1364.

Hendricks WM. Sudden appearance of multiple kera-toacanthomas three weeks after thermal burn. *Cutis*. 1991;47:410–412.

Herchline TE, Ayers LW. Occurrence of *Staphylococcus lugdunensis* in consecutive clinical cultures and rela-tionship of isolation to infection. *J Clin Microbiol*. 1991;29:419–421.

Herzog A. Dangerous errors in the diagnosis and treatment of bony tuberculosis. *Ditsch Arziebl Int*. 2009;106:573–577.

Hoke CH Jr, Batt JM, Mirrett S, et al. False-positive Gram-stained smears. *JAMA*. 1979;241:471–480.

Homer MJ, Aguilar-Delfin I, Telford SR III, et al. Babesiosis. *Clin Microbiol Rev*. 2000;13:451–469.

Hope WW, Walsh TJ, Denning DW. Laboratory diagnosis of invasive aspergillosis. *Lancet Infect Dis*. 2005;5:609–622.

Horsburgh CR Jr. Disseminated infection with *Mycobacterium avium-intracellulare*. *Medicine*. 1985;64:36–48.

Hughes R, McGuire G. Delayed diagnosis of disseminated strongyloidiasis. *Intensive Care Med.* 2001;27:310–312.

Hunt DP, Thabet A, Rosenberg ES. Case records of the Massachusetts General Hospital. Case 29-2010: a 29-year-old woman with fever and abdominal pain. *N Engl J Med.* 2010;363:1266–1274.

Hurt C, Tammaro D. Diagnostic evaluation of mononucleosis-like illnesses. *Am J Med.* 2007;120:e1–e8.

Hutter RV. The surgical pathologist as a diagnostician and consultant. *Am J Clin Pathol.* 1981;75(suppl 3):447–452.

Ibrarullah M, Mohan A, Sarkari A, et al. Abdominal tuberculosis: diagnosis by laparoscopy and colonoscopy. *Trop Gastroenterol.* 2002;23:150–153.

Igra-Siegman Y, Kapila R, Sen P, et al. Syndrome of hyperinfection with *Strongyloides stercoralis. Rev Infect Dis.* 1981;3:397–407.

Inaba AS, Zukin DD, Perro M. An update on the evaluation and management of plantar puncture wounds and *Pseudomonas* osteomyelitis. *Pediatr Emerg Care.* 1992;8:38–44.

Ingram CW, Tanner DC, Durack DT, et al. Disseminated infection with rapidly growing mycobacteria. *Clin Infect Dis.* 1993;16:463–471.

Isaacs D. Problems in determining the etiology of community-acquired childhood pneumonia. *Pediatr Infect Dis J.* 1989;8:143–148.

Jaakkola J, Kehl D. Hematogenous calcaneal osteomyelitis in children. *J Pediatr Orthop.* 1999;19:699–704.

Jacob CN, Henein SS, Heurich AE, Kamholz S. Nontuberculous mycobacterial infection of the central nervous system in patients with AIDS. *South Med J.* 1993;86:638–640.

Jadavji T, Law B, Lebel MH, et al. A practical guide for the diagnosis and treatment of pediatric pneumonia. *CMAJ.* 1997;156(suppl):S703–S711.

Jaggers J, Balsara K. Mediastinal masses in children. *Semin Thorac Cardiovasc Surg.* 2004;16:201–208.

Johansson N, Kalin M, Tiveljung-Lindell A, et al. Etiology of community-acquired pneumonia: increased microbiological yield with new diagnostic methods. *Clin Infect Dis.* 2010;50:202–209.

Jones O, Cleveland KO, Gelfand MS. A case of disseminated histoplasmosis following autologous stem cell transplantation for Hodgkin's lymphoma: an initial misdiagnosis with a false-positive serum galactomannan assay. *Transpl Infect Dis.* 2009;11:281–283.

Kahn JO, Walker BD. Acute human immunodeficiency virus type 1 infection. *N Engl J Med.* 1998;339:33–39.

Kain KC, Harrington MA, Tennyson S, Keystone JS. Imported malaria: prospective analysis of problems in diagnosis and management. *Clin Infect Dis.* 1998;27:142–149.

Kapoor H, Signs K, Somsel P, et al. Persistence of West Nile virus (WNV) IgM antibodies in cerebrospinal fluid from patients with CNS disease. *J Clin Virol.* 2004;31:289–291.

Karakelides H, Aubry MC, Ryu JH. Cytomegalovirus pneumonia mimicking lung cancer in an immunocompetent host. *Mayo Clin Proc.* 2003;78:488–490.

Kathir K, Dennis C. Primary pulmonary botryomycosis: an important differential diagnosis for lung cancer. *Respirology.* 2001;6:347–350.

Katsuya H, Takata T, Ishikawa T, et al. A patient with acute myeloid leukemia who developed fatal pneumonia caused by carbapenem-resistant *Bacillus cereus. J Infect Chemother.* 2009;15:39–41.

Kaufmann JM, Zaenglein AL, Kaul A, Chang MW. Fever and rash in a 3-year-old girl: Rocky Mountain spotted fever. *Cutis.* 2002;70:165–168.

Kerleguer A, Fabre M, Bernatas JJ, et al. Clinical evaluation of the Gen-Probe Amplified *Mycobacterium tuberculosis* Direct Test for rapid diagnosis of tuberculosis lymphadenitis. *J Clin Microbiol.* 2004;42:5921–5922.

Khan R, Abid S, Jafn W, et al. Diagnostic dilemma of abdominal tuberculosis in non-HIV patients: an ongoing challenge for physicians. *World J Gastroenterol.* 2006;12:6371–6375.

Kieslich M, Fiedler A, Driever PH, et al. Lyme borreliosis mimicking central nervous system malignancy: the diagnostic pitfall of cerebrospinal fluid cytology. *Brain Dev.* 2000;22:403–406.

Kirchner SG, Hernanz-Schulman M, Stein SM, et al. Imaging of pediatric mediastinal histoplasmosis. *Radiographics.* 1991;11:365–381.

Kleiner E, Monk AB, Archer GL, Forbes BA. Clinical significance of *Staphylococcus lugdunensis* isolated from routine cultures. *Clin Infect Dis.* 2010;51:801–803.

Korownyk C, Allan GM. Evidence-based approach to abscess management. *Can Fam Physician*. 2007;53:1680–1684.

Kratz A, Laposata M. Enhanced clinical consulting—moving toward the core competencies of laboratory professionals. *Clin Chim Acta*. 2002;319:117–125.

Kristoferitsch W. Neurological manifestations of Lyme borreliosis: clinical definition and differential diagnosis. *Scand J Infect Dis Suppl*. 1991;77:64–73.

Kyriacou DN, Spira AM, Talan DA, Mabey DC. Emergency department presentation and misdiagnosis of imported *falciparum* malaria. *Ann Emerg Med*. 1996;27:696–699.

Lachance DH, O'Neill BP, Macdonald DR, et al. Primary leptomingeal lymphoma: report of 9 cases, diagnosis with immunocytochemical analysis, and review of the literature. *Neurology*. 1991;41:95–100.

Lahti E, Peltola V, Waris M, et al. Induced sputum in the diagnosis of childhood community-acquired pneumonia. *Thorax*. 2009;64:252–257.

Lambert AJ, Nasci RS, Cropp BC, et al. Nucleic acid amplification assays for detection of La Crosse virus RNA. *J Clin Microbiol*. 2005;43:1885–1889.

Lang CM, Hofmann WP, Kriener S, et al. Primary actinomycosis of the liver mimicking malignancy. *Z Gastroenterol*. 2009;47:1062–1064.

Laposata M. Patient-specific narrative interpretation of complex clinical laboratory evaluations: who is competent to provide them? *Clin Chem*. 2004;50:471–472.

Larkin JA, Shashy RG, Gonzalez CA. Difficulty in differentiating a rapidly growing *Mycobacterium* species from diphtheroids in an immunocompromised patient. *Clin Microbiol Newsl*. 1997;19:108–111.

Lazcano O, Speights VO Jr, Stickler JG, et al. Combined histochemical stains in the differential diagnosis of *Cryptococcus neoformans*. *Mod Pathol*. 1993;6:80–84.

Leape LL, Woods DD, Hatlie MJ, et al. Promoting patient safety by preventing medical error. *JAMA*. 1998;280:1444–1447.

Lecour H, Miranda M, Margo C, et al. Human leptospirosis—a review of 50 cases. *Infection*. 1989;17:8–12.

Lee CW, Lim MJ, Son D, et al. A case of cerebral gumma presenting as brain tumor in a human immunodeficiency virus (HIV)-negative patient. *Yonsei Med J*. 2009;50:284–288.

Lee IK, Liu JW. Osteomyelitis concurrently caused by *Staphylococcus aureus* and *Mycobacterium tuberculosis*. *South Med J*. 2007;100:903–905.

Lee K, Chong Y, Shin HB, et al. Modified Hodge and EDTA-disk synergy tests to screen metallo-beta-lactamase-producing strains of *Pseudomonas* and *Acinetobacter* species. *Clin Microbiol Infect*. 2001;7:88–91.

Lee SY, Kwon HJ, Cho JH, et al. Actinomycosis of the appendix mimicking appendiceal tumor: a case report. *World J Gastroenterol*. 2010;16:395–397.

Lefmann M, Moter A, Schweickert B, Gobel UB. Misidentification of *Mycobacterium leprae* as *Mycobacterium intracellulare* by the COBAS AMLICOR *M. intracellulare* Test. *J Clin Microbiol*. 2005;43:1928–1929.

Li JY, Lo ST, Ng CS. Molecular detection of *Mycobacterium tuberculosis* in tissues showing granulomatous inflammation without demonstrable acid-fast bacilli. *Diagn Mol Pathol*. 2009;9:67–74.

Lippi G, Banfi G, Buttarello M, et al. Recommendations for detection and management of unsuitable samples in clinical laboratories. *Clin Lab Chem Med*. 2007;45:728–736.

Lippi G, Blanckaert N, Bonini P, et al. Causes, consequences, detection, and prevention of identification errors in laboratory diagnosis. *Clin Chem Lab Med*. 2009;47:143–153.

Lippi G, Guidi GC. Risk management in the preanalytic phase of laboratory testing. *Clin Chem Lab Med*. 2007;45:720–727.

Lippi G, Guidi GC, Mattiuzzi C, Plebani M. Pre-analytical variability: the dark side of the moon in laboratory testing. *Clin Chem Lab Med*. 2006;44:358–365.

Liu PY, Huang YF, Tang CW, et al. *Staphylococcus lugdunensis* infective endocarditis: a literature review and analysis of risk factors. *J Microbiol Immunol Infect*. 2010;43:478–484.

Lo A, Verrall R, Williams J, et al. Carbapenem resistance via the bla_{KPC-2} gene in *Enterobacter cloacae* blood culture isolate. *South Med J*. 2010;103:394–395.

Lo Re V III, Gluckman SJ. Fever in the returned traveler. *Am J Fam Physician*. 2003;68:1343–1350.

Lopez Martinez L, Mendez Tovar LJ. Chromoblastomycosis. *Clin Dermatol*. 2007;25:188–194.

Lundberg GD. When to panic over abnormal values. *MLO Med Lab Obs*. 1972;4:47–54.

Lundberg GD. Critical (panic) value notification: an established laboratory policy (parameter). *JAMA*. 1990;263:709.

Lundberg GD. Is it time to extend the laboratory critical (panic) value system to include vital values? *MedGenMed*. 2007;9:20.

Luzuriaga K, Sullivan JL. Infectious mononucleosis. *N Engl J Med*. 2010;362:1993–2000.

Madhusudhan KS, Gamanagatti S, Seith A, Hari S. Pulmonary infections mimicking cancer: report of four cases. *Singapore Med J*. 2007;48:e327–e331.

Malane MS, Grant-Keis JM, Feder HM Jr, Lugar SW. Diagnosis of Lyme disease based on dermatologic manifestation. *Ann Intern Med*. 1991;114:490–498.

Mandell LA, Wunderlink RG, Anzueto A, et al. Infectious Diseases Society of America/American Thoracic Society consensus guidelines on the management of community-acquired pneumonia in adults. *Clin Infect Dis*. 2007;44(suppl 2):S27–S72.

Mantur BG, Malimani MS, Bidari LH, et al. Bacteremia is as unpredictable as clinical manifestations in human brucellosis. *Int J Infect Dis*. 2008;12:303–307.

Marchevsky AM, Damsker B, Green S, Tepper S. The clinicopathological spectrum of non-tuberculous mycobacterial osteoarticular infections. *J Bone Joint Surg*. 1985;67(6):925–929.

Martin GS, Christman BW, Standaert SM. Rapidly fatal infection with *Ehrlichia chaffeensis*. *N Engl J Med*. 1999;341:763–764.

Martin WJ. Rapid and reliable techniques for the laboratory detection of bacterial meningitis. *Am J Med*. 1983;75:119–123.

Massie RJ, Van Asperen PP, Mellis CM. A review of open biopsy for mediastinal masses. *J Paediatr Child Health*. 1997;33:230–233.

Masters EJ, Olson GS, Weiner SJ, Paddock CD. Rocky Mountain spotted fever: a clinician's dilemma. *Arch Intern Med*. 2003;163:769–774.

Mattei D, Rapezzi D, Mordini N, et al. False-positive *Aspergillus* galactomannan enzyme-linked immunosorbent assay result *in vivo* during amoxicillin-clavulanic acid treatment. *J Clin Microbiol*. 2004;42:5262–5263.

Mazuchowski EL II, Meier PA. The modern autopsy: what to do if infection is suspected. *Arch Med Res.* 2005;36:713–723.

McCabe RE, Brooks RG, Dorfman RF, Remington JS. Clinical spectrum in 107 cases of toxoplasmic lymphadenopathy. *Rev Infect Dis.* 1987;9:754–774.

Meijer JAA, Sjogren EV, Kuijper E, et al. Necrotizing cervical lymphadenitis due to disseminated *Histoplasma capsulatum* infection. *Eur J Clin Microbiol Infect Dis.* 2005;24:574–576.

Mennink-Kersten MA, Donnelly JP, Verweij PE. Detection of circulating galactomannan for the diagnosis and management of invasive aspergillosis. *Lancet Infect Dis.* 2004;4:349–357.

Mennink-Kersten MA, Warris A, Verweij PE. 1,3-β-D-glucan in patients receiving intravenous amoxicillin-clavulanic acid. *N Engl J Med.* 2006;354:2834–2835.

Miller EH, Semian DW. Gram-negative osteomyelitis following puncture wounds of the foot. *J Bone Joint Surg Am.* 1975;57:535–537.

Molecular identification of pathogenic fungi. *J Antimicrob Chemother.* 2008;61(suppl 1):S7–S12.

Molloy PJ, Persing DH, Berardi VP. False-positive results of PCR testing for Lyme disease. *Clin Infect Dis.* 2001;33:413–414.

Muder RR, Yu BL. Infection due to *Legionella* species other than *L. pneumophila*. *Clin Infect Dis.* 2002;35:990–998.

Muller SA, Vogt P, Altwegg M, Seebach JD. Deadly carousel or difficult interpretation of new diagnostic tools for Whipple's disease: case report and review of the literature. *Infection.* 2005;33:39–42.

Muneef MA, Memish Z, Mohmoud SA, et al. Tuberculosis in the belly: a review of forty-six cases involving the gastrointestinal tract and peritoneum. *Scand J Gastroenterol.* 2001;36:528–532.

Murdoch DR. Diagnosis of *Legionella* infection. *Clin Infect Dis.* 2003;36:64–69.

Musher DM, Montoya R, Wanahita A. Diagnostic value of microscopic examination of Gram-stained sputum and sputum cultures in patients with bacteremic pneumococcal pneumonia. *Clin Infect Dis.* 2004;39:165–169.

Musher DM, Schell RF. Letter: false-positive Gram stains of cerebrospinal fluid. *Ann Intern Med*. 1973;79:603–604.

Narreddy S, Chandrasekar PH. False-positive *Aspergillus* galactomannan (GM) assay in histoplasmosis. *J Infect*. 2008;56:80–81.

Nenoff P, Kellermann S, Borte G, et al. Pulmonary nocardiosis with cutaneous involvement mimicking a metastasizing lung carcinoma in a patient with chronic myelogenous leukaemia. *Eur J Dermatol*. 2000;10:47–51.

Neuman MI, Tolford S, Harper MB. Test characteristics and interpretation of cerebrospinal fluid Gram stain in children. *Pediatr Infect Dis J*. 2008;27:309–313.

Newberry AM, Williams DN, Stauffer WM, et al. *Strongyloides* hyperinfection presenting as acute respiratory failure and gram-negative sepsis. *Chest*. 2005;128:3681–3684.

Newton HJ, Ang DKY, van Driel IR, Hartland EL. Molecular pathogenesis of infections caused by *Legionella pneumophila*. *Clin Microbiol Rev*. 2010;23:274–298.

Noble MA. Developments in external quality assessment for clinical microbiology laboratories. *Accred Qual Assur*. 2004;9:601–604.

O'Brien D, Tobin S, Brown GV, Torresi J. Fever in returned travelers: a review of hospital admissions for a 3-year period. *Clin Infect Dis*. 2001;33:603–609.

Odio CM, Navarrete M, Carrillo JM, et al. Disseminated histoplasmosis in infants. *Pediatr Infect Dis J*. 1999;18:1065–1068.

Olivier R, Godfroid E, Heintz R, et al. Lyme borreliosis in a patient with severe multiple cranial neuropathy. *Clin Infect Dis*. 1995;20:200.

O'Reilly M, Paddock C, Elchos B, et al. Physician knowledge of the diagnosis and management of Rocky Mountain spotted fever: Mississippi, 2002. *Ann N Y Acad Sci*. 2003;990:295–301.

Ostrosky-Zeichner L, Alexander BD, Kett DH, et al. Multicenter clinical evaluation of the $(1{\rightarrow}3)$-β-D-glucan assay as an aid to diagnosis of fungal infections in humans. *Clin Infect Dis*. 2005;41:654–659.

Ozaki T, Nishimura N, Arakawa Y, et al. Community-acquired *Acinetobacter baumannii* meningitis in a previously healthy 14-month-old boy. *J Infect Chemother*. 2009;15:322–324.

Ozdemir H, Tapisiz A, Ciftei E, et al. Successful treatment of three children with post-neurosurgical multidrug-resistant *Acinetobacter baumannii* meningitis. *Infection.* 2010;38:241–244.

Ozturk R, Mert A, Kocak F, et al. The diagnosis of brucellosis by use of BACTEC 9240 blood culture system. *Diagn Microbiol Infect Dis.* 2002;44:133–135.

Parola P, Raoult D. Ticks and tickborne bacterial diseases: an emerging infectious threat. *Clin Infect Dis.* 2001;32: 897–926.

Patel R, Grogg KL, Edwards WD, et al. Death from inappropriate therapy for Lyme disease. *Clin Infect Dis.* 2000;31:1107–1109.

Patterson JW. An extracellular body of plasma cell origin in inflammatory infiltrates within the dermis. *Am J Dermatopathol.* 1986;8:117–123.

Peacock SJ, Schweizer HP, Dance DA, et al. Management of accidental laboratory exposure to *Burkholderia pseudomallei* and *B. mallei. Emerg Infect Dis.* 2008;14:e2.

Peleg AY, Seifert H, Paterson DL. *Acinetobacter baumannii:* emergence of a successful pathogen. *Clin Microbiol Rev.* 2008;21:538–582.

Penn RL, Normand R, Klotz SA. Factitious meningitis: a recurring problem. *Infect Control Hosp Epidemiol.* 1988;9:501–503.

Persing DH. Polymerase chain reaction: trenches to benches. *J Clin Microbiol.* 1990;29:1281–1285.

Pershing DH, Mathiesen D, Marshall WF, et al. Detection of *Babesia microti* by polymerase chain reaction. *J Clin Microbiol.* 1992;30:2097–2103.

Peterson L, Thrupp L, Uchiyama N, et al. Factitious bacteria meningitis revisited. *J Clin Microbiol.* 1982;16:758–760.

Pitrak DL, Koneman EW, Estupinan RC, Jackson J. *Phialophora richardsiae* infection in humans. *Rev Infect Dis.* 1988;10:1195–1203.

Plouffe JF, File TM, Breiman RF, et al. Reevaluation of the definition of Legionnaires' disease: use of the urinary antigen assay; Community Based Pneumonia Incidence Study Group. *Clin Infect Dis.* 1995;20:1286–1291.

Poirel L, Nordmann P. Carbapenem resistance in *Acinetobacter baumannii:* mechanisms and epidemiology. *Clin Microbiol Infect.* 2006;12:826–836.

Powers CN. Diagnosis of infectious diseases: a cytopathologist's perspective. *Clin Microbiol Rev.* 1998;11:341–365.

Prince HE, Calma J, Pham T, Seaton BL. Frequency of missed cases of probable acute West Nile virus (WNV) infection when testing for WNV RNA alone or WNV immunoglobulin M alone. *Clin Vaccine Immunol.* 2009;16: 587–588.

Prince LK, Shali AA, Martinez LJ, Moran KA. Ehrlichiosis: making the diagnosis in the clinical setting. *South Med J.* 2007;100:825–828.

Quireshi MZ, New D, Zulgarni NJ, Nachman S. Overdiagnosis and overtreatment of Lyme disease in children. *Pediatr Infect Dis.* 2002;21:12–14.

Rand KH, Tillan M. Errors in interpretation of Gram stains from positive blood cultures. *Am J Clin Pathol.* 2006;126:686–690.

Raoult D, Birg M, La Scola B, et al. Cultivation of the bacillus of Whipple's disease. *N Engl J Med.* 2000;342:620–625.

Recommendations for test performance and interpretation from the Second National Conference on Serologic Diagnosis of Lyme Disease. *MMWR Morb Mortal Wkly Rep.* 1995;44:590–591.

Reiss E, Miller SE, Kaplan W, Kaufman L. Antigenic, chemical, and structural properties of cell walls of *Histoplasma capsulatum* yeast-form chemotypes 1 and 2 after serial enzymatic hydrolysis. *Infect Immun.* 1977;16:690–700.

Reiss E, Mitchell WO, Stone SH, Hasenclever HF. Cellular immune activity of a galactomannan-protein complex from mycelia of *Histoplasma capsulatum. Infect Immun.* 1974;10:802–809.

Reiss E, Obayashi T, Orle K, et al. Non-culture based diagnostic tests for mycotic infections. *Med Mycol.* 2000;38(suppl 1):147–159.

Repath F, Seabury JH, Sanders CV, Domer J. Prosthetic valve endocarditis due to *Mycobacterium chelonei. South Med J.* 1976;69:1244–1246.

Ricaldi JN, Vinetz JM. Lepatospirosis in the tropics and in travelers. *Curr Infect Dis Rep.* 2006;8:51–58.

Robboy SJ. The clinical pathologist: physician, not administrator. *Hum Pathol.* 1982;13:788–789.

Roberts FJ. Procurement, interpretation, and value of postmortem cultures. *Eur J Clin Microbiol Infect Dis.* 1998;17:821–827.

Robichaud S, Libman M, Behr M, Rubin E. Prevention of laboratory-acquired brucellosis. *Clin Infect Dis.* 2004;38:e119–e122.

Rolain JM, Lepidi H, Zanaret M, et al. Lymph node biopsy specimens and diagnosis of cat-scratch disease. *Emerg Infect Dis.* 2006;12:1338–1344.

Rolston KV, Rodriguez S, Dholakia N, et al. Pulmonary infections mimicking cancer; a retrospective, three-year review. *Support Care Cancer.* 1997;5:90–93.

Rosenberg ES, Callendo AM, Walker BD. Acute HIV infection among patients tested for mononucleosis. *N Engl J Med.* 1990;340:969.

Rosenbloom ST, Stead WW, Denny JC, et al. Generating clinical notes for the electronic health record systems. *Appl Clin Inform.* 2010;1:232–243.

Rossi SL, Ross TM, Evans JD. West Nile virus. *Clin Lab Med.* 2010;30:47–65.

Ryan ET, Wilson ME, Kain KC. Illness after international travel. *N Engl J Med.* 2002;347:505–516.

Saccente M, Woods GL. Clinical and laboratory update on blastomycosis. *Clin Microbiol Rev.* 2010;23:367–381.

Saha DC, Xess I, Jain N. Evaluation of conventional & serological methods for rapid diagnosis of cryptococcus. *Indian J Med Res.* 2008;127:483–488.

Samant S, Sandoe J, High A, Makura ZG. Actinomycosis mimicking a tonsillar neoplasm in an elderly diabetic patient. *Br J Oral Maxillofac Surg.* 2009;47:417–418.

Samuels MA, Newell KL. Case records of the Massachusetts General Hospital. Case 32-1997. A 43-year-old woman with rapidly changing pulmonary infiltrates and markedly increased intracranial pressure. *N Engl J Med.* 1997;337:1149–1156.

Sandhu G, Ranade A, Ramsinghani P, Noel C. Influenza-like illness as an atypical presentation of *falciparum* malaria in a traveler from Africa. *J Emerg Med.* 2011;41:35–38.

Sanford CC. Puncture wounds of the foot. *Am Fam Physician.* 1981;24:119–122.

Sangoi AR, Rogers WM, Longacre TA, et al. Challenges and pitfalls of morphologic identification of fungal infections in histologic and cytologic specimens: a ten-year retrospective review at a single institution. *Am J Clin Pathol.* 2009;13:364–375.

Schwartz J. The diagnosis of deep mycoses by morphologic methods. *Hum Pathol*. 1982;13:519–533.

Schwetschenau E, Kelly DL. The adult neck mass. *Am Fam Physician*. 2002;66:831–838.

Scott M. Infections involving lymph nodes. In: Collins RD, Swerdlow SH, eds. *Pediatric Hematopathology*. Philadelphia, PA: Churchill Livingstone; 2001:289.

Seabolt JP. *Babesia*: challenges for the medical technologist. *Lab Med*. 1982;13:547–551.

Seenivasan MH, Yu VL. *Staphylococcus lugdunensis* endocarditis—the hidden peril of coagulase-negative staphylococcus in blood cultures. *Eur J Clin Microbiol Infect Dis*. 2003;22:489–491.

Segarra-Newnham M. Manifestations, diagnosis, and treatment of *Strongyloides stercoralis* infection. *Ann Phamacother*. 2007;41:1992–2001.

Sehouli J, Stupin JH, Schlieper U, et al. Actinomycotic inflammatory disease and misdiagnosis of ovarian cancer: a case report. *Anticancer Res*. 2006;26:1727–1731.

Seifert H. The clinical importance of microbiological findings in the diagnosis and management of bloodstream infections. *Clin Infect Dis*. 2009;48(suppl):S238–S245.

Setty S, Khalil Z, Schori P, et al. Babesiosis. Two atypical cases from Minnesota and a review. *Am J Clin Pathol*. 2003;120:554–559.

Shah M, Centor RM, Jennings M. Severe acute pharyngitis caused by group C streptococcus. *J Gen Intern Med*. 2007;22:272–274.

Sharp SE, Elder BL. Competency assessment in the clinical microbiology laboratory. *Clin Microbiol Rev*. 2004;17:681–694.

Shorman M, Al-Tawfiq JA. *Strongyloides stercoralis* hyperinfection presenting as acute respiratory failure and gram-negative sepsis in a patient with astrocytoma. *Int J Infect Dis*. 2009;13:e288–e291.

Sigal LH. Pitfalls in the diagnosis and management of Lyme disease. *Arthritis Rheum*. 1998;41:195–204.

Signori C, Ceriotti F, Messeri G, et al. Process and risk analysis to reduce errors in clinical laboratories. *Clin Chem Lab Med*. 2007;45:742–748.

Sikora M, Interewicz B, Olszewski WL. Contemporary methods for detection of microbial infections in transplanted tissues. *Ann Transplant*. 2005;10:11–16.

Simons CM, Stratton CW, Kim AS. Peripheral blood eosinophilia as a clue to the diagnosis of an occult *Coccidioides* infection. *Hum Pathol.* 2011;42:449–453.

Simpson J, Campbell PE. Mediastinal masses in childhood: a review from a paediatric pathologist's point of view. *Prog Pediatr Surg.* 1991;27:92–126.

Sinnott JT IV, Cancio MR, Frankle MA, Spiegel PG. Tuberculous osteomyelitis masked by concomitant staphylococcal infection. *Arch Intern Med.* 1990;150:1865–1867.

Sivalingam SK, Saligram P, Natanasabapathy S, Paez A. Covert cryptococcal meningitis in a patient with systemic lupus erythematous. *J Emerg Med.* 2014;47:323–325.

Smallman LA, Young JA, Shortland-Webb WR, et al. *Strongyloides stercoralis* hyperinfection syndrome with *Escherichia coli* meningitis: report of two cases. *J Clin Pathol.* 1986;39:366–370.

Smith MB, Boyars MC, Woods GL. Fatal *Mycobacterium fortuitum* meningitis in a patient with AIDS. *Clin Infect Dis.* 1996;23:1327–1328.

Smith MB, Schnadig VJ, Boyars MC, Woods GL. Clinical and pathologic features of *Mycobacterium fortuitum* infections. An emerging pathogen in patients with AIDS. *Am J Clin Pathol.* 2001;116:225–232.

Sokol DK, Kleiman MB, Garg BP. LaCrosse viral encephalitis mimics herpes simplex viral encephalitis. *Pediatr Neurol.* 2001;25:413–415.

Somsouk M, Shergill AK, Grenert JP, et al. Actinomycosis mimicking a pancreatic head neoplasm diagnosed by EUS-guided FNA. *Gastrointest Endosc.* 2008;68:186–187.

Son YM, Kang HK, Na SY, et al. Chromoblastomycosis caused by *Phialophora richardsiae*. *Ann Dermatol.* 2010;22:362–366.

Sotutu V, Carapetis J, Wilkinson J, et al. The "surreptitious *Staphylococcus*": *Staphylococcus lugdunensis* endocarditis in a child. *Pediatr Infect Dis J.* 2002;21:984–986.

Southern PM Jr, Colvin DD. Pseudomeningitis again. Association with cytocentrifuge funnel and Gram-stain reagent contamination. *Arch Pathol Lab Med.* 1996;120:456–458.

Spagnuolo PJ, Fransioli M. Intrauterine device–associated actinomycosis simulating pelvic malignancy. *Am J Gastroenterol.* 1981;75:144–147.

Sperber SJ, Schleupner CJ. Leptospirosis: a forgotten cause of aseptic meningitis and multisystem febrile illness. *South Med J.* 1989;10:1285–1288.

Spratt BG, Cromie KD. Penicillin-binding proteins of gram-negative bacteria. *Rev Infect Dis.* 1988;10:699–711.

Srinivasan J, Ooi WW. Successful treatment of histoplasmosis brain abscess with voriconazole. *Arch Neurol.* 2008;65:666–667.

Stead WW. Electronic health records. *Stud Health Technol Inform.* 2010;153:119–143.

Steere AC, Taylor E, McHugh GL, Logigian EL. The overdiagnosis of Lyme diease. *JAMA.* 1993;269:1812–1816.

Stefaniuk E, Baraniak A, Gniadkowski M, Hryniewicz W. Evaluation of the BD Phoenix automated identification and susceptibility testing system in clinical microbiology practice. *Eur J Clin Microbiol Infect Dis.* 2003;22:479–485.

Strand CL. Positive blood cultures: can we always trust the Gram stain? *Am J Clin Pathol.* 2006;126:671–672.

Stratton CW. Susceptibility testing today. Myth, reality, and new direction. *Hosp Epidemiol.* 1988;9:264–267.

Stratton CW. *In vitro* susceptibility testing versus *in vivo* effectiveness. *Med Clin North Am.* 2006;90:1077–1088.

Suarez JI, Mlakar D, Snodgrass SM. Cerebral syphilitic gumma in an HIV-negative patient presenting as prolonged focal motor status epilepticus. *N Engl J Med.* 1996;335:1159–1160.

Sugiura Y, Homma M, Yamamoto T. Difficulty in diagnosing chronic meningitis caused by capsule-deficient *Cryptococcus neoformans. J Neurol Neurosurg Psychiatry.* 2005;76:1460–1461.

Suh KN, Kozarsky PE, Keystone JS. Evaluation of fever in the returned traveler. *Med Clin North Am.* 1999;83:997–1017.

Sulahian A, Touratier S, Ribaud P. False positive test for *Aspergillus* antigenemia related to concomitant administration of piperacillin and tazobactam. *N Engl J Med.* 2003;349:2366–2367.

Surani S, Chandra H, Weinstein RA. Breast abscess: coagulase-negative staphylococcus as a sole pathogen. *Clin Infect Dis.* 1993;17:701–704.

Tacoveanu E, Dimofte G, Bradea C, et al. Peritoneal tuberculosis in laparoscopic era. *Acta Chir Belg.* 2009;109:65–70.

Takahashi N, Shimada T, Ishibashi Y, et al. The pitfall of coagulase-negative staphylococci: a case of *Staphylococcus lugdunensis* endocarditis. *Int J Cardiol*. 2009;137:e15–e17.

Taylor TH, Albrecht MA. *Legionella bozemanii* cavitary pneumonia poorly responsive to erythromycin: case report and review. *Clin Infect Dis*. 1995;20:329–334.

Theerthakarai R, Al-Halees W, Ismail M, et al. Nonvalue of the initial microbiological studies in the management of nonsevere community-acquired pneumonia. *Chest*. 2001; 119:5–7.

Thompson AJ, Brown MM, Ridley A. *Escherichia coli* meningitis and disseminated strongyloidiasis. *J Neurol Neurosurg Psychiatry*. 1988;51:1596–1597.

Thomson RB Jr, Peterson LR. Role of the clinical microbiology laboratory in the diagnosis of infections. *Cancer Treat Res*. 1998;96:143–165.

Thomson RB Jr, Wilson ML, Weinstein MP. The clinical microbiology laboratory director in the Unities States hospital setting. *J Clin Microbiol*. 2010;48:3465–3469.

Tilley PAG, Fox JD, Jayaraman GC, Preiksaitis JK. Nucleic acid testing for West Nile virus RNA in plasma enhances rapid diagnosis of acute infection in symptomatic patients. *J Infect Dis*. 2006;193:1361–1364.

Timmermans M, Carr J. Neurosyphilis in the modern era. *J Neurol Neurosurg Psychiatry*. 2004;75:1727–1730.

To KK, Cheng VC, Tang BS, et al. False-negative cerebrospinal fluid cryptococcal antigen test due to small-colony variants of *Cyrptococcus neoformans* meningitis in a patient with cystopleural shunt. *Scand J Infect Dis*. 2006;38: 1110–1114.

Trevenzoli M, Sattin A, Sgarabotto D, et al. Splenic infarct during infectious mononucleosis. *Scand J Infect Dis*. 2001;33:550–551.

Trumbull ML, Chesney TM. The cytological diagnosis of pulmonary blastomycosis. *JAMA*. 1981;245:836–838.

Tsai WC, Hsieh HC, Su HM, et al. *Mycobacterium abscessus* endocarditis: a case report and literature review. *Kaohsiung J Med Sci*. 2008;24:481–486.

Tugwell P, Dennis DT, Weinstein A, et al. Laboratory evaluation in the diagnosis of Lyme disease. *Ann Intern Med*. 1997;127:1109–1123.

Tunkel AR, Hartman BJ, Kaplan SL, et al. Practice guidelines for the management of bacterial meningitis. *Clin Infect Dis*. 2004;391:1267–1284.

Uyeki TM, Prasad R, Bukotich C, et al. Low sensitivity of rapid diagnostic tests for influenza. *Clin Infect Dis*. 2009;48:e89–e92.

Uyeki TM, Sharma A, Branda JA. Case records of the Massachusetts General Hospital. Case 40-2009. A 29-year-old man with fever and respiratory failure. *N Engl J Med*. 2009;36:2558–2569.

Uzunkoy A, Harma M, Harma M. Diagnosis of abdominal tuberculosis: experience from 11 cases and review of the literature. *World J Gastroenterol*. 2004;10:3647–3649.

Vance DW. Group C streptococci: "*Streptococcus equisimilis*" of *Streptococcus anginosus*? *Clin Infect Dis*. 1992;14:616.

Van Hoovels L, De Munter P, Colaert J, et al. Three cases of destructive native valve endocarditis caused by *Staphylococcus lugdunensis*. *Eur J Clin Microbiol Infect Dis*. 2005;24:149–152.

Vannier E, Gewurz BE, Krause PJ. Human babesiosis. *Infect Dis Clin N Am*. 2008;22:469–488.

Vassilakopoulos TP, Pangalis GA. Application of a prediction rule to select which patients presenting with lymphadenopathy should undergo a lymph node biopsy. *Medicine (Baltimore)*. 1996;79:338–347.

Vijayachari P, Sugunan AP, Shriram AN. Leptospirosis: an emerging global public health problem. *J Biosci*. 2008;33:557–569.

Von Graevenitz A, Punter-Streit V. Failure to recognize rapidly growing mycobacteria in a proficiency testing sample without specific request: a wider diagnostic problem? *Eur J Epidemiol*. 1998;14:519–520.

Wadei H, Alangaden GJ, Sillix DH, et al. West Nile virus encephalitis: an emerging disease in renal transplant recipients. *Clin Transplant*. 2004;18:753–758.

Waghorn DJ. *Staphylococcus lugdunensis* as a cause of breast abscess. *Clin Infect Dis*. 1994;19:814–815.

Wallace RJ, Swenson JM, Silcox VA, et al. Spectrum of disease due to rapidly growing mycobacteria. *Rev Infect Dis*. 1983;5:657–679.

Walther EU, Seelos K, Bise K, et al. Lyme neuroborreliosis mimicking primary CNS lymphoma. *Eur Neurol.* 2004;5:43–45.

Weber CL, Bartley D, Al-Thaqafi A, Embil JM. *Blastomyces dermatitidis* osteomyelitis of the tibia. *Am J Orthop.* 2007;36:29–32.

Weesner CL, Cisek JE. Lemierre syndrome: the forgotten disease. *Ann Emerg Med.* 1993;22:256–258.

Weinstein RA, Bauer FW, Hoffman RD, et al. Factitious meningitis. Diagnostic error due to nonviable bacteria in commercial lumbar puncture trays. *JAMA.* 1975;233:878–879.

Weissert C, Dollenmaier G, Rafeiner P, et al. *Burkholderia pseudomallei* misidentified by automated system. *Emerg Infect Dis.* 2009;15:1799–1801.

Wernaers P, Handelberg F. Brucellar arthritis of the knee: a case report with delayed diagnosis. *Acta Orthop Belg.* 2007;73:795–798.

Werno AM, Murdoch DR. Laboratory diagnosis of invasive pneumococcal disease. *Clin Infect Dis.* 2008;46:926–932.

Wheat LJ, Kohler RB, Tewari RP. Diagnosis of disseminated histoplasmosis by detection of *Histoplasma capsulatum* antigen in serum and urine specimens. *N Engl J Med.* 1986;314:83–88.

Whiley RA, Hall LM, Hardie JM, Beighton D. A study of small-colony, beta-haemolytic, Lancefield group C streptococci within the *anginosus* group: description of *Streptococcus constellatus* subsp. pharyngitis subsp. nov., associated with the human throat and pharyngitis. *Int J Syst Bacteriol.* 1999;49(pt 4):1433–1439.

Whipple GH. A hitherto undescribed disease characterized anatomically by deposits of fat and fatty acids in the intestinal and mesenteric lymphatic tissues. *Bull Johns Hopkins Hosp.* 1907;18:382–391.

Widmer A, Hohl P, Dirnhofer S, et al. *Legionella bozemanii*, an elusive agent of fatal cavitary pneumonia. *Infection.* 2007;35:180–181.

Wiersinga WJ, van der Poll T, White NJ, et al. Melioidosis insights into the pathogenicity of *Burkholderia pseudomallei. Nat Rev Microbiol.* 2006;4:272–282.

Williamson JC, Miano TA, Morgan MR, Palavecino EL. Fatal *Mycobacterium abscessus* endocarditis misidentified as *Corynebacterium* spp. *Scand J Infect Dis.* 2010;42:222–224.

Wilson ML, Winn W. Laboratory diagnosis of bone, joint, soft-tissue, and skin infections. *Clin Infect Dis.* 2008;46:453–457.

Witte DA, Chen I, Brady J, et al. Cryptococcal osteomyelitis. Report of a case with aspiration biopsy of a humeral lesion with radiologic features of malignancy. *Acto Cytol.* 2000;44:815–818.

Wolfert AL, Wright JE. Whipple's disease presenting as sarcoidosis and valvular heart disease. *South Med J.* 1999;92:820–825.

Woods GL, Walker DH. Detection of infection or infectious agents by use of cytologic and histologic stains. *Clin Microbiol Rev.* 1996;9:382–404.

Woods WG, Singher LJ, Krivit W, Nesbit ME Jr. Histoplasmosis simulating lymphoma in children. *J Pediatr Surg.* 1979;14:423–425.

Wormser GP. Early Lyme disease. *N Engl J Med.* 2006;354:2794–2801.

Wurtz R, Paleologos N. LaCrosse encephalitis presenting like herpes simplex encephalitis in an immunocompromised adult. *Clin Infect Dis.* 2000;31:1284–1287.

Yamazaki Y, Kitagawa Y, Hata H, et al. Cervical toxoplasmic lymphadenitis can mimic malignant lymphoma on FDG PET. *Clin Nucl Med.* 2008;33:819–820.

Yangco BG, TeStrake E, Okafor J. *Phialophora richardsiae* isolated from infected human bone: morphological, physiological and antifungal susceptibility studies. *Mycopathologia.* 1984;86:103–111.

Zeharia A, Eidlitz-Markus T, Haimi-Cohen Y, et al. Management of nontuberculous mycobacteria-induced cervical lymphadenitis with observation alone. *Pediatr Infect Dis J.* 2008;27:920–922.

CHAPTER 6
Laboratory Management

CANDIS A. KINKUS

ACCREDITATION AND REGULATORY COMPLIANCE

Laboratory services are regulated at the federal level, and in many cases, by one or more state agencies as well. If state regulations are more stringent than federal, then the state regulations supersede federal. In addition, there are federally designated, nongovernment agencies that conduct periodic and unannounced on-site inspections of laboratories. These inspections serve to document performance compliance with standards and thereby accredit the laboratory to receive or maintain a federal license to operate. This federal license is referred to as a "Clinical Laboratory Improvement Amendments (CLIA)" license as laboratory licensure was deemed a regulatory requirement with the enactment of the CLIA of 1988.

Good management requires that the leadership team understand both the federal and state laws as well as the accreditation standards established by the inspecting agencies. It is the leadership team's responsibility to ensure that actual laboratory practice complies with both legal regulations and accreditation requirements. Failure to do so may lead to consequences ranging from almost nothing to the catastrophic for the laboratory service: for example, from a substandard performance that requires a repeat inspection to unacceptable performance with suspension of license and testing.

UNDERSTAND REQUIREMENTS OF STATE REGULATIONS

The management team must be aware of government (federal, state, and local) regulations, accreditation standards, and institutional policies. These performance requirements apply to a broad range of laboratory activities, including personnel, safety, reports and records, claims billing, and waste disposal.

PREPARE FOR INSPECTION

Unannounced inspection for licensure is a routine practice. At a moment's notice, the laboratory management team must produce numerous test procedures and quality report records that demonstrate performance over a two-year period. This requires a standard practice for documenting and maintaining records of test and instrument performance, quality control, written procedures, and reviews, so that these can be readily produced at the time of inspection.

COLLABORATE WITH INSTITUTIONAL DEPARTMENTS

There are accreditation standards and regulations that define key data elements that must appear on a test results report. However, the laboratory test report is also a medicolegal record. As such, all test results and comments are subject to interpretation in any legal proceeding.

STANDARDS OF PERFORMANCE

- Laboratory management should verify and understand regulatory requirements at all levels of government: federal, state, and local. Federal regulations, including CLIA, routinely state that the federal requirements are a minimum performance standard and do not supersede more stringent standards from state and local government agencies. It is also important to know the performance standards for any other regulatory agency, such as the College of American Pathologists, The Joint Commission, and the American Association of Blood Banks, that has accreditation oversight of the laboratory. The laboratory's procedures and policies must meet the most stringent requirements imposed by the applicable regulatory entity or accrediting agency.

▦ While laboratory inspectors arrive unannounced, they are fully prepared and expect to complete all aspects of inspection within a specific time frame for that site. It is imperative that the management team has defined a standard process for maintaining necessary and complete documents and records, so that these can be readily produced at the time of inspection.

▦ The laboratory test result report is a medicolegal document and this applies to all information contained on the report, not just the test results. Statements that are simple and clear in everyday communication may not meet those legal standards in a court of law. As test result reports are created or revised, the management team is responsible for ensuring that these documents are properly reviewed and approved.

PATIENT SAFETY

The Institute of Medicine report published in 2000 clearly documented an unacceptable number of negative outcomes for patients. One of the key factors contributing to the problems in patient care is the failure of health care providers to define safe practice standards and consistently enforce compliance. This report led to the development of the patient safety standards by numerous agencies, including The Joint Commission and the College of American Pathologists.

A key patient safety standard for the laboratory is to ensure positive patient identification (PPID). It is a required practice that PPID must use two unique patient identifiers. These identifiers usually include the patient's complete name and one or more of the following: medical record number, complete birth date, or Social Security number. Once a specimen has been received in the laboratory and is in process, a common practice is to assign a unique accession number that may be used in conjunction with the patient's name during the testing process.

The PPID practice is a critical step in the preanalytic phase of laboratory testing. Some accrediting agencies require that at the time of specimen collection, health care providers must use both "active and passive" identification methods. Passive identification requires the health care provider to verify the printed patient identifiers (on specimen labels, test requisitions, or computer screen) with a patient identification armband that must be attached to the wrist or ankle of an admitted patient. For active identification, the employee is required to engage the patient to verbally confirm his or her identity. A common practice is to request the patient to state his or her complete name, spell his or her last name, and provide his or her complete date of birth. The employee must verify that the patient's responses match the printed identifiers (on specimen labels, test requisitions, or computer screen).

During the analytic phase, many test methods require manual processes. It is necessary to design workflow to ensure that the patient identity is correctly maintained with the specimen throughout testing.

Likewise, in the postanalytic phase, there are some circumstances that may warrant providing a verbal result to the clinician. It is imperative that this communication between both parties occurs with the use of PPID.

Regardless of the accuracy of the test method, a correct result provided for the wrong patient can have dire consequences, including loss of life. Laboratory leadership is responsible for defining clear procedures for patient safety, training staff to ensure competency, and consistently maintaining accountability for compliance by all staff at all times.

PERFORM PROPER SPECIMEN COLLECTION

When performing PPID, the phlebotomist often has multiple computer-generated labels that will be applied to each test tube. It is necessary to verify the patient identifiers on each printed label, not just on the first label.

In the outpatient setting, patients present for specimen collection, but do not receive a patient identification armband. However, the patient does have a physician's written test order with the patient's complete name. A common practice is to use this document in lieu of the identification band. When performing passive and active patient identification, it is incumbent upon the phlebotomist to verify all computer-generated labels and the patient's verbal identification with the written test order.

In addition to performing both passive and active patient identification, another requirement of PPID is to label all specimen containers at the patient's side. This practice minimizes the risk of error that a label could inadvertently be applied to a specimen collected from another patient.

VERIFY PATIENT IDENTIFICATION IN THE ANALYTIC PHASE

Many test methods require that an aliquot of the specimen be manually transferred from the original specimen container to another container (tube, well, plate, cassette) for testing. It is absolutely necessary to verify the patient identification on the original specimen container with the patient identification on the test container. Standard procedure is to perform this specimen transfer process on a one-by-one basis. The employee should only work with one patient at a time when transferring specimens from one container to another. This practice reduces the risk of erroneously transferring a sample from one patient to a container identified for another patient.

To minimize the amount of blood collected from a patient, it is common practice to use one tube of blood or body fluid for tests that are performed in multiple departments. The usual practice is to properly label new test containers and then aliquot samples from the original specimen. Patient identifiers on the original tube and aliquot tubes should be verified as the samples are dispensed.

If the initial test result is positive and the method requires a repeat test to validate an original positive result, it is recommended to obtain the original specimen container, if possible, and perform the repeat test with a sample from the original specimen container.

The importance of performing specimen transfer on a one-by-one basis cannot be overemphasized. It is analogous to the patient safety standard that requires that all specimen containers are labeled at the patient's side. Both of these practice standards are intended to ensure that the specimen material in the container actually belongs to the patient identified on the container.

CONFIRM PATIENT IDENTITY WHEN PROVIDING VERBAL RESULTS

In the vast majority of patient care situations, information technology enables the clinician to have ready electronic access to test results. However, there are circumstances where a patient is in critical condition and the provider does not have immediate electronic access to results. The clinician will then call the laboratory and request a verbal report of *the results. At any given time, the laboratory is performing tests on dozens if not hundreds of patients. Patients with the same or very similar names can be undergoing testing in the same time frame. It is still necessary to obtain patient identifiers to ensure that the correct results will be provided on the correct patient.*

STANDARDS OF PERFORMANCE

■ The laboratory service is unlike any other health care service in that testing is performed in the absence of the patient. Thus, it is absolutely imperative to define procedures to ensure that both patients and patients' specimens are accurately identified throughout the testing process. Staff must consistently comply with key performance standards for PPID.

■ At the time of collection, a health care provider must perform both active and passive identification. In those circumstances where the patient cannot communicate, the laboratory should define appropriate actions in consultation with risk management. All labels must be applied to specimen containers in the presence of the patient.

■ During the analytic phase, it is particularly important to design manual work processes to minimize the risk of erroneously placing patient specimens in an incorrectly labeled test container.

■ All verbal communication must include unique patient identifiers. This will reduce the risk of confusing information about two different patients with the same or similar names.

QUALITY MANAGEMENT AND PERFORMANCE IMPROVEMENT

A defined quality management (QM) program is an essential tool to measure the success of clinical testing services. A QM program must evaluate the production of test results across the entire performance spectrum: the preanalytic stage, the analytic stage, and the postanalytic stage.

The clinical leadership is responsible for identifying specific performance indicators to monitor against defined performance thresholds. Generally, tests are selected for monitoring based on the potential impact to patient care. "High volume" tests are those for which errors would affect a large number of patients. "High risk" tests are those for which errors would produce serious negative outcomes, including loss of life or limb. Performance indicators should include appropriate activities across the preanalytic, analytic, or postanalytic phases.

Performance thresholds may be defined in several ways. A common practice is to base a threshold on the required outcomes for patient care, such as a turnaround time (TAT) of 40 minutes for test results ordered on stroke patients for whom timely therapeutic drug intervention is required. Some performance benchmarks are determined by the accreditation standards, for example, the presence of two unique patient identifiers on specimen containers.

There are some tests that largely serve an outpatient population. In this setting, it is necessary to understand the industry standards established in the commercial marketplace such as acceptable wait times for patients in an outpatient phlebotomy service.

COLLECT AND ANALYZE DATA TO SUPPORT PATIENT OUTCOMES

To effectively evaluate routine performance of a test at any phase, one must first measure the activity and then define the performance standard. It is often necessary to conduct several observations and measure the time to complete the procedure from start to finish. Once the performance standard is determined, then the performance threshold can be defined. Generally, an acceptable performance threshold is reported as the ability of the laboratory to complete the procedure and meet the performance standard with a high rate of success. A poorly defined performance threshold or inadequate data collection will lead to a failure to identify problems with the procedure, and thereby pose an undue risk to patient care.

DEFINE PERFORMANCE STANDARDS

When there is a failure to accurately define a performance standard, then it will not be possible to identify problems and take corrective action. Various performance indicators can be monitored such as the TAT for test results or patient wait times. A threshold must be appropriately defined for each performance indicator. The actual performance can then be compared to the threshold and evaluated as to whether the actual performance is acceptable or unacceptable.

STANDARDS OF PERFORMANCE

- Laboratory performance must be measured to ensure that the service meets or exceeds the defined standard. An appropriate performance threshold must be defined for the performance indicator.
- Measuring performance indicators requires that a representative sample must be collected for data analysis. Therefore, it is necessary to understand the unique characteristics that are associated with a particular test or procedure.
- It is important to consider the most applicable unit of measure when reporting a performance indicator. Many accrediting agencies frequently define acceptable performance as the ability to meet the performance standard at least 80% of the time.
- Generally, reporting an absolute number for performance indicators is an appropriate measure to

use where errors can have significant consequences such as an incorrect blood transfusion.

FINANCIAL MANAGEMENT

Provision of laboratory services requires resources: staff, equipment, and supplies. The leadership is responsible for acquiring resources and managing expenses in both the operating and capital budgets. It is also necessary to manage the revenue stream so that billing claims are submitted correctly and timely to maximize payment for services.

When assessing the expansion of an existing laboratory service or implementation of new test programs, the financial impact of the operating costs (if necessary, capital expenses as well) must be calculated. This financial analysis should also consider other factors. The opportunity cost of not choosing to pursue new or expanded programs must be assessed. This evaluation should include the impact on patient care such as a decreased length of stay (LOS) by decreasing result TAT. A financial assessment should also consider the pros and cons of "make versus buy" and determine whether it is cheaper and more efficient to "make" the test in the laboratory or "buy" it from a vendor.

Operating expenses should be routinely monitored on a monthly basis. Supervisory staff should review budget reports for actual expenses and confirm that both staff salary and supply costs are correct. It is important to engage staff so that they can contribute to controlling supply expense. Employees should understand that payment for services is not provided until 45 days or more from the date when the claim is submitted. Defined processes for inventory management should be structured to minimize unnecessary overstocking on supplies.

Conversely, billable test volume and revenues must be regularly reviewed as well. Management oversight should include verification that the correct Current Procedural Terminology (CPT) codes are submitted on claims. The timeliness of claim submissions should be monitored as well to minimize the risk of nonpayment for services rendered.

MONITOR SUPPLY EXPENSES

Supply inventory should be managed so that reasonable quantities are maintained on site. Excessive supply inventory ties up financial resources that could be better spent on salaries, capital equipment purchase, new or expanded programs, and infrastructure needs.

The management team must routinely review actual expenses that are charged to the operating budget. Although much of the purchasing and accounts payable functions are electronically processed, there are still opportunities for error.

MANAGE REVENUE

In those few situations when a new test method is released with a new CPT code, it is important to verify that insurers will reimburse payment for the new test. However, there are circumstances when an existing test with a CPT code will be recommended as part of a new protocol for patient care diagnosis or treatment. This situation also warrants a review to determine that insurers will reimburse payment for the new use of the test.

Managers should use financial reporting tools to monitor the revenue cycle. A commonly used report is one that monitors the number of denied claims. This report can indicate problems that require the manager to investigate and take action to ensure that payments are received. Claims may be denied due to delays in submitting claims, incorrect CPT codes or modifiers, missing or incorrect diagnosis, and many other causes.

ASSESS PROGRAM OPPORTUNITIES

When evaluating the financial impact of a test, the potential effect on patient care must be considered as well. Upon initial examination, a test may have a modest financial impact on the laboratory budget. However, the results may allow providers to initiate treatment so that it substantially benefits both patient care and the institution's financial picture.

STANDARDS OF PERFORMANCE

- Managers should routinely monitor supply expense and inventory. In addition, all laboratory staff must participate in effectively managing supplies to better control operating expenses. For every dollar in operating cash spent on supplies, one dollar less is available for salaries and capital equipment.
- The need to obtain the best price for supplies should be balanced with maintaining a reasonable inventory. Generally, payment for testing services is not received until 45 days or longer after the service has been performed. Thus, there is little benefit to investing operating cash to purchase a product that could last for many months or years.
- Operating budget reports should be reviewed monthly to ensure that appropriate supply expenses are documented. This includes verifying that all lease payments or reagent rental fees are correct, as per the contracts.
- Product inventory should be monitored and this includes those test supply items that are provided to clients. For those supplies that are provided to clients, there should be a reasonable association between the test volumes returned to the laboratory with supply items delivered to the client.
- Operational processes should support accurate and timely billing and claims submission to ensure that the full revenue payment is received for services

rendered. When implementing new test programs it may be necessary to confirm that insurers will provide reimbursement for a new service.

- Automated electronic billing must be used as new tests are added to the test order menu. This will ensure that claims are consistently and correctly submitted within contractual requirements.
- Financial management reports should be monitored to identify any problems with claims submissions and payment denials. The manager is responsible for taking corrective action to ensure that claims are accurate, complete, and meet contractual deadlines.
- The laboratory leadership is responsible for recognizing the larger impact of the laboratory service on patient care. There may be circumstances when incurring additional costs to provide a laboratory service is more than offset by an enhanced outcome for patient care.

STAFF MANAGEMENT

The laboratory leadership is responsible for ensuring that qualified staff are hired and properly trained to provide accurate test results. Building a team of competent employees starts with the proper selection of candidates.

A well-defined training program is necessary to ensure consistent performance by all new employees. Orientation training must also include competency assessments to objectively measure actual task performance relative to the procedure standard.

Management must also define and communicate objective performance standards to staff. Employees should receive periodic reports so that they can clearly understand how they are completing their work as compared with the standard.

SELECT QUALIFIED CANDIDATES

The selection process starts with a well-defined job description that includes required education, experience, and skills. It is necessary to interview candidates and thoroughly assess their capabilities to meet the job requirements. However, it is equally important to evaluate the candidate's interpersonal communication skills with other employees and to obtain objective references from the candidate's current and previous employers.

DEFINE STANDARDS AND MEASURE ACTUAL PERFORMANCE

Performance standards should be clearly defined and communicated to staff so that they understand what is required to successfully accomplish tasks. It also enables coworkers to form a stronger sense of team since their work is measured based on objective standards and not subjective perception.

ADDRESS COMPENSATION ISSUES

Many factors can impact the ability to hire and retain staff. A competitive salary is one of the key elements for attracting and retaining employees. Laboratory management must identify those circumstances that can create a noncompetitive position with salaries. It is also important to engage the human resources staff to assist with collecting data and, if necessary, finding solutions.

ASSESS STAFFING LEVELS AND WORKLOAD

It is important to monitor test volume activity and identify when new staff are required. This allows the laboratory to continue to meet performance standards and minimize any disruption in service.

STANDARDS OF PERFORMANCE

▓ Evaluating candidates should include an assessment of their clinical expertise and their communication and interpersonal skills. When possible, candidates should be interviewed by colleagues and subordinates as well as by superiors.

▓ It is recommended that references are obtained from both current and previous employers when an applicant is the preferred candidate for a position.

▓ Clearly define objective and quantifiable performance measures for employees. This allows employees to understand what is expected and enables the laboratory to dependably support patient care.

▓ Identify conditions in the marketplace that can affect salaries and impact an employer's competitive position. The human resources staff can provide the necessary data to justify appropriate actions to recruit and retain staff.

▓ Monitor test activity to determine staffing needs. When appropriate, analyze data and define when staffing coverage should be assigned.

LABORATORY SAFETY

The laboratory leadership team must ensure that the work environment complies with safety standards as defined by government regulations, accreditation standards, and institutional policies. In addition to implementing procedures, the staff must be educated to properly perform safety procedures and comply with them.

DEFINE PROCEDURES AND MONITOR COMPLIANCE

Since the mid-1980s, the Occupational Safety and Health Administration (OSHA) has required that personal protective equipment must be used in all situations where there is a risk of biohazard exposure. In the laboratory, all staff are required to wear laboratory coats and gloves when handling specimens and performing tests.

Laboratory management must have defined written procedures for laboratory safety and must monitor compliance with these procedures. Staff are required to comply with all safety procedures, and laboratory leadership is responsible for holding staff accountable to properly perform work in accordance with the safety standards.

STANDARDS OF PERFORMANCE

▧ Laboratory management is obligated to implement defined procedures that meet safety requirements and monitor staff compliance with safety standards. Appropriate staff resources within the laboratory and from outside departments should be actively engaged with defining, implementing, and monitoring laboratory safety matters.

▧ Safety practices are applicable to all employees who perform those tasks that are covered by government regulations or institutional policies. As new safety initiatives are implemented, staff should be trained in proper practice and understand that there are consequences for noncompliance. It is management's responsibility to monitor compliance and provide a mechanism to allow staff to report safety failures without fear of retaliation.

SPECIMEN LOGISTICS

An important step in the preanalytic process is the transport and delivery of specimens to the laboratory bench. It is imperative to understand the regulations that govern specimen transport and ensure that the actual practice is in compliance. The transport process must be designed to minimize the risk of losing specimens as they are moved from the collection site to the laboratory bench.

There are Department of Transportation regulations that define numerous standards for transporting biohazardous materials. These regulations apply to both internal transport within the hospital from the patient "bedside" to the laboratory and external transport by courier services from an outside facility to the laboratory. A health care facility is accountable for contracted vendors. Therefore, it is incumbent upon the laboratory management to ensure that its contract with an outside courier service requires vendor compliance with regulations. The laboratory will be liable should a contracted courier service fail to meet Department of Transportation standards.

There should also be an efficient process to ensure that specimens are moved from the collection site to the laboratory bench. This process should be designed to move the specimens in a timely manner. Within a health care facility, it is generally easy to accomplish timely transport through the use of pneumatic tube transport systems. The widespread adoption of computerized provider order entry enables the laboratory to better manage pending test orders with the receipt of patient specimens. However, this process design is more challenging when moving specimens from satellite collection facilities to the laboratory.

TRANSPORT SPECIMENS FROM SATELLITE SITES

Specimens must be transported, at all times, in a manner that complies with all safety standards and minimizes risk of exposure to biohazardous materials. A process for "handing off" specimens from one location to another must be defined for both routine and nonroutine circumstances. Any number of communication tools (verbal, written, or electronic) can be appropriately applied to the situation in an effort to minimize the risk of losing specimens.

DEFINE EFFICIENT WORKFLOW PROCESS

Workflow should be designed so that staff can complete tasks with consistent efficiency. When possible, nonvalue-added tasks should be removed from the work process.

STANDARDS OF PERFORMANCE

▦ All specimen transport activities must comply with government regulations to ensure that there is minimal risk of biohazardous exposure or contamination. Laboratories are responsible to ensure that both their employees and contracted vendors acceptably perform these duties.

▦ The procedure for transporting specimens should be designed to ensure that there is documentation of a specimen's location as it moves through the "transport system." Documentation can be either electronic or paper and, when necessary, may need to include verbal communication as well.

▦ The workflow process should be efficiently designed to move the specimen from the preanalytic step to the bench for analysis. Nonvalue-added tasks should be removed and reassigned to designated staff.

TEST UTILIZATION

In the ongoing national debate concerning the growing consumption of health care services, increased expenditures for laboratory tests, particularly molecular diagnostics, face continued scrutiny to control costs. Evaluating test utilization should cover both inpatient and outpatient activity as well as those tests that are performed in the laboratory and those sent to an outside vendor.

Effectively managing test utilization produces both operational and financial benefits. By reducing excessive orders for tests, there is available capacity, with both staff and instruments, to implement new tests as the need arises and to absorb increased volume. It will also increase the net revenue margin for test services that are reimbursed through capitated payments.

CREATE PARTNERSHIPS WITH KEY CLIENTS

In its effort to appropriately manage test orders, the laboratory leadership should consider engaging external resources. These resources can include practicing physicians who are "thought leaders" within a medical specialty, information technology tools that can monitor activity, or consultative expertise from other areas such as finance, compliance, legal, or risk management.

MANAGE TEST UTILIZATION

Inappropriate utilization of some tests may occur because there is a poor understanding of the appropriate clinical indications. The laboratory clinical leaders can actively manage appropriate test utilization and constructively support the providers.

STANDARDS OF PERFORMANCE

- Patient care providers can obtain large amounts of diagnostic information from numerous tests. Whenever appropriate, the laboratory leadership should engage technology to assist in appropriately directing the selection and ordering of tests.
- Laboratory management must be effective stewards of its employees, instruments, and supplies. Test order patterns should be periodically monitored to

identify any excessive or unnecessary utilization. Appropriate test order activity will ensure that laboratory resources are efficiently supporting patient care and that there is available capacity to manage increased volume and implement new tests.

COMPETITIVE PERFORMANCE IN THE OUTREACH MARKET

Hospital laboratories have long recognized the opportunities of testing services in the outpatient market. The hospital has the capital infrastructure and capacity in the off-hour shifts that coincidentally is the time frame when most outreach testing is performed. A hospital laboratory also has an existing relationship with the physicians who admit patients and can build on that relationship.

Hospital laboratory leadership must recognize that performance standards in the outreach market are decidedly different from those for their inpatients. To succeed in outreach, the hospital laboratory must compete with commercial laboratories and at least meet, if not exceed, the performance standards in the outpatient marketplace. It is imperative to understand the service standards, conduct a SWOT (strengths, weaknesses, opportunities, and threats) analysis, and implement the necessary processes to meet the clients' service expectations.

UNDERSTAND SERVICE REQUIREMENTS

The laboratory management team often attempts to capitalize on its "strength" of clinical expertise. Frequently though, the laboratory fails to adequately evaluate the clients' service needs or provide the clinical consultation most needed by the ordering physician.

MANAGE STAFF PERFORMANCE TO SUPPORT OUTREACH MARKET

There are many service demands in the outreach market that do not coincide with service demands for inpatients and hospital unit staff. It is incumbent upon the laboratory leadership to understand the outreach service requirements, educate the staff, and implement any necessary workflow changes to support the clients' service needs.

DEFINE INFRASTRUCTURE REQUIREMENTS

Hospital laboratories can engage support for the outreach market from a broad array of services provided by other departments such as finance and marketing. It is management's responsibility to constructively engage colleagues in other departments and clearly communicate service needs and to assist with development and implementation.

STANDARDS OF PERFORMANCE

- Once the specific laboratory services for the outreach market have been identified, it is imperative to evaluate the service requirements as defined by the clients. Service requirements can be very broadly defined from ease of test ordering and availability of specimen collection supplies to complete and comprehensive reports that are consistently delivered in a timely manner.
- Management must ensure that there are adequate resources, both instrument and staff, so that clients' service needs are reliably met.
- The management team must educate staff to understand that the service needs for the "outreach" market are different, and problems must be appropriately addressed. When there is a failure at any step in the process (preanalytic, analytic, or postanalytic phases), there should be a defined procedure

that directs staff to notify the appropriate individuals who can assist with troubleshooting and problem resolution.

Competing in the "outreach" market often requires infrastructure support outside of traditional hospital laboratory operations. The laboratory manager must enlist key departments, such as finance, IT, and marketing, and engage them so that they fully understand the performance requirements to meet the clients' service needs. Laboratory leadership should maintain constructive and ongoing communication with these external departments so that they can continue to support the service demands for the "outreach" clients.

SELECTION AND MANAGEMENT OF REFERENCE LABORATORIES

The volume of tests sent to reference laboratories generally comprises a relatively small percentage of total ordered tests. However, the expenses incurred for reference laboratory services often constitute a significant portion of the supply budget. With the introduction of molecular diagnostic tests, the costs for reference laboratory testing have been growing exponentially for more than a decade. Laboratory leadership must be actively engaged in the selection of vendors for reference testing service and the providers' utilization of this resource.

MONITOR UTILIZATION OF REFERENCE LABORATORIES

For hospital-based laboratories, there are regulatory requirements that stipulate that the selection of reference laboratories must be determined jointly by the laboratory leadership and the hospital's medical staff. It is necessary for laboratory leadership to actively engage in the selection and use of reference laboratory facilities. The laboratory management team possesses the expertise to carefully evaluate the clinical quality, suitability of the test menu to meet patient needs, and service performance of the various vendors. These factors, in addition to cost, must be assessed when selecting a reference laboratory.

EVALUATE VENDORS' FULL SCOPE OF PERFORMANCE

Given the explosive growth in molecular testing, managers are finding that costs for reference testing can consume 10% or more of total supply costs. It is certainly essential to consider costs when evaluating vendors for reference laboratory testing. However, clinical quality and service performance must also be considered. The vendor must meet defined clinical and service criteria so that the patient care needs are appropriately provided. Also, regulatory requirements hold the hospital laboratory accountable for any subcontractor's performance.

STANDARDS OF PERFORMANCE

- Even when a contract is in place with a vendor, the cost for reference testing can spiral out of control when providers are given carte blanche to both order tests and select the reference testing site. Laboratory leadership must monitor "leakage" of tests to noncontracted vendors and, where appropriate, engage the clinicians and redirect the tests.
- Common business practice does require a competitive bid for those services that incur significant expense. However, the selection of a reference laboratory service should be evaluated on clinical performance and service requirements as well as cost. Consideration of these three elements can better ensure that the necessary diagnostic needs for patient care are addressed in addition to the business need to effectively control costs.

INSTRUMENT SELECTION FOR THE CLINICAL LABORATORY

The diagnostic laboratory industry is composed of manufacturers who compete in both the national and global marketplace. There are a large number of instruments available to meet the needs of both commercial and hospital-based laboratories of all sizes. It is imperative to clearly understand patient care needs in order to properly select instruments. Selection criteria should include clinical method evaluation, reagent stability, throughput capacity, ease of use and process control, and documented instrument performance and vendor service record.

UNDERSTAND PATIENT CARE NEEDS

The acquisition of any major instrument requires a thorough consideration of both current patient care needs and any new programs. Failure to do so may create a situation where the laboratory is unable to properly support patient care needs over the life of the instrument.

EVALUATE COMPETITIVE PRODUCTS

Many laboratory instruments are offered by manufacturers who compete in the global marketplace. As in any industry, these competitive forces drive manufacturers to continuously enhance their instruments and reagents. Laboratory management should engage in a competitive evaluation of products to ensure that it is providing the latest technology that best meets patient care needs and optimizes the efficient use of resources.

STANDARDS OF PERFORMANCE

■ The acquisition of new instrument technology must consider the current and future patient care needs. Laboratory managers should collaborate with key departments, such as finance, business development, and marketing, to identify programs planned for future implementation that will require support from the new instrument. Clearly defining current and anticipated patient testing needs can improve the instrument selection process by providing for discounted costs triggered by volume targets and enhanced performance requirements from the vendor.

▦ An instrument reaching the end of its useful life presents an opportunity to comparatively assess new technology and select an instrument and reagent system that can best support patient care. Many instruments have a useful life of 5 to 7 years or sometimes more. However, the competitive forces in the marketplace drive technological innovations during that same period of time. These innovations can benefit patient care and laboratory operations and should be evaluated.

▦ Clinical performance is crucial to evaluating instruments. However, many other factors must be considered as well. Methods should be assessed to ensure that staff can work efficiently and in a manner that minimizes the risk of errors. The financial assessment should identify "hidden" costs that may be associated with quality control, instrument maintenance, or other factors such as a renovation expense that may be required for installation.

SELECTION AND UTILIZATION OF A LABORATORY INFORMATION SYSTEM

The laboratory information system (LIS) represents a strategic investment in data management capabilities and capital funds. These laboratory test results provide essential information to providers for the diagnosis and treatment of patients in both inpatient and outpatient settings. Therefore, the selection and ongoing operation of an LIS requires participation from a broad array of users, clients, and key stakeholders.

When selecting an LIS, the users, both pathologists and technologists, must identify performance requirements such as capabilities for managing and processing test orders, interfacing with various instruments and other software information systems, manipulation of data to support numerous requirements for results reporting, and supporting ancillary functions such as billing, client services and QM, and process control. A dedicated team from across the clinical and anatomical pathology services should define and rank the performance requirements. These criteria can serve as an objective tool to evaluate each LIS application.

Laboratory clients include physicians and nurses. They may have test order or result report needs for patient care that should be considered when assessing LIS applications.

Key stakeholders include other departments that must interact on some level with the LIS. For example, the information technology group provides services such as network support or interface design and maintenance associated with other software applications. Finance is another department that may rely on the LIS for obtaining coding data and completing claims submission. It is necessary to engage these key stakeholders and assure that the LIS will not compromise any necessary operational processes with external departments.

Lastly, the management team must understand the level of staff expertise that is required to support the LIS, including adequate staff coverage and the necessary training of users.

DETERMINE STAFF SUPPORT FOR LIS

The laboratory leadership should manage the LIS installation so that its performance is optimized to support data management. When extensive custom modifications are required for the software, management should understand and plan for the necessary support resources.

CONFIRM COMPATABILITY WITH OTHER SOFTWARE APPLICATIONS

There are a number of software applications that must be interfaced to an LIS. The "owners" of these external information systems should participate in evaluating the new LIS products to ensure that there is an acceptable degree of compatibility. Failure to do so can create unnecessary problems.

SUPPORT CLIENTS' SERVICE EXPECTATIONS

Periodically, a laboratory will expand its test menu. When providing a new service, it is important to understand the service requirements that clients may have for these result reports.

STANDARDS OF PERFORMANCE

▨ It is the responsibility of laboratory leadership to understand and define the resources required to support the LIS. Resource needs can vary depending on the complexity of the LIS. A highly customized LIS will require staff with programming expertise, whereas a simple "turnkey" application will require vendor-trained staff.

▨ The LIS provides critical support for data management of test orders and results. Given the laboratory's key role in patient diagnosis and treatment, it is absolutely essential that the LIS can effectively communicate with various independent software applications. The laboratory leadership is responsible for engaging key stakeholders of external software applications and ensuring that all necessary performance requirements can be met.

- When selecting a new LIS, a laboratory team should be formed with representation from across numerous subspecialties. The team should define and prioritize performance requirements that can then be used as an objective tool to measure capabilities of various LIS applications.
- Clients' needs for test ordering or result reporting should be solicited. They should be engaged when evaluating a new LIS and also when there is a service update.

BIBLIOGRAPHY

A number of textbooks are available that can provide a more extensive discussion of management concepts and practices that are applicable to the laboratory setting. The following is a brief list of resources for the interested reader:

Garcia LS, ed. *Clinical Laboratory Management.* Washington, DC: ASM Press; 2004.

Harmening D. *Laboratory Management: Principles and Processes.* 2nd ed. Philadelphia, PA: FA Davis; 2007.

Hudson J. *Principles of Clinical Laboratory Management: A Study Guide and Workbook.* Upper Saddle River, NJ: Prentice Hall; 2003.

Lewandrowski K, ed. *Clinical Chemistry Laboratory Management and Clinical Correlations.* Philadelphia, PA: Lippincott Williams & Wilkins; 2002.

O'Brien JA. *Common Problems in Clinical Laboratory Management.* New York, NY: McGraw-Hill; 1999.

Varnadoe LA. *Medical Laboratory Management and Supervision: Operations, Review and Study Guide.* Philadelphia, PA: FA Davis; 1996.

Index

"abnormal platelet distribution"
    flag, 131
ABO system, 11–12
absolute lymphocytosis, 127
absolute reticulocyte counts, 125
accreditation
    laboratory management, 259
    standards and
        regulations, 260
ACE-i. *See* angiotensin-
    converting enzyme
    inhibitors
acetaminophen, 37, 38
acetone, 213
Acinetobacter baumannii, 212
Acinetobacter species, 213
ACOG. *See* American Congress
    of Obstetricians and
    Gynecologists
ACPA tests. *See* anticitrullinated
    peptide antibody tests
active clotting, 97–98
active identification, 262, 263, 265
acute clinical management, 155
acute HIV-1 infection, 226
acute West Nile encephalitis, 198
ADAMTS 13 assays, 110, 111
adverse events, transfusion of
    FFP, 1
albumin, 15
alert values. *See* critical values
allogeneic blood, transfusion
    of, 12
alloimmune thrombocytopenia
    in primigravida, risk of,
    48–49

American Association of Blood
    Banks (AABB), 4, 6
American Congress of
    Obstetricians and
    Gynecologists (ACOG), 4
amniotic fluid bilirubin level,
    33, 34
analytical errors
    in clinical microbiology, 210
    core chemistry, 149–151
    endocrine testing, 174
    laboratory information
        systems, 176–177
    point-of-care testing, 166–169
    therapeutic drug monitoring/
        toxicology, 152–153
anaphylactic transfusion
    reaction, 34, 35
anaphylaxis, 35
anaplasmosis, 194
ANCA. *See* antineutrophil
    cytoplasmic antibodies
ANCA-associated vasculitides
    (AAVs), 134
anemia, errors in diagnosis of,
    123–124
angiotensin-converting
    enzyme inhibitors (ACE-i),
    36, 37
anti–beta-2 glycoprotein I
    antibodies, 101
antibody-antigen reaction, 23
antibody detection, 11
anticardiolipin antibodies, 101
anticitrullinated peptide
    antibody (ACPA) tests, 134

anticoagulant-associated
  intracerebral hemorrhage
  (AAICH), 31
anticoagulant therapy
  monitoring
  in patients with argatroban, 76
  in patients with
    fondaparinux, 72–73
  in patients with low
    molecular weight
    heparin, 67–68
  in patients with
    unfractionated heparin,
    63–64
  in patients with warfarin, 59
anti-factor Xa assay
  fondaparinux, 73, 74
  low molecular weight
    heparin, 68, 69
  unfractionated heparin, 64–66
antigenic tests, 136
antigen typing, 11
anti-IgA antibody, 34
anti-Kell alloantibodies, 33–34
antineutrophil cytoplasmic
  antibodies (ANCA) tests,
  errors in interpretation of,
  134–135
antinuclear antibody tests,
  errors in interpretation of,
  131–132
antiphospholipid antibodies,
  evaluation for, 100
antiplatelet agents, platelet
  dysfunction evaluation
  in, 114
antithrombin
  in active clotting, 97
  antigenic tests for, 95
  in children, 97
  deficiency of, 96
apheresis platelets, 24
approval-only ordering, 186
argatroban
  anticoagulant therapy
    monitoring in patients
    with, 76

clot-based activated protein C
    resistance assay, 94
  coagulation factor assays, 85
aspirin
  baseline platelet function, 114
  platelet transfusion for
    patients on, 24–25
atypical lymphocytosis,
    differential diagnosis
    of, 127
autoimmune, immunology, 131
autologous blood, inappropriate
    use of, 12–13
automated control process, 147
automated electronic
    billing, 271

babesiosis, 196
Bacillus cereus, 212
Bacillus infections, 212
BCC. *See Burkholderia cepacia*
    complex
BCYE agar. *See* buffered charcoal
    yeast extract agar
beta-lactamases, 212
Bethesda unit, factor VIII
    inhibitor, 109
biopsy, 192
Blastomyces dermatitidis, 215
blind operators, 166–167
blood, 11
    circulation, exposure to,
    17–18
    issue of, 8–9
    transfusion, refusal of, 27–28
blood collection, 208
blood donors, adverse reactions
    in, 28–29
blood sample collection, error
    in, 9–10
blood sample for anti-factor Xa
    monitoring, 70
B lymphocytes, blastoid
    transformation of, 197
bone marrow aspirations, 192
bone marrow biopsy, 128
Borrelia, 200

Borrelia burgdorferi infection, 197
broad-spectrum empirical antimicrobial therapy, 198
bronchoscopy specimens, 202
buffered charcoal yeast extract (BCYE) agar, 202
Burkholderia cepacia complex (BCC), 216
Burkholderia pseudomallei, 216

CAD. *See* cold agglutinin disease
CA-MRSA. *See* Community-associated methicillin-resistant Staphylococcus Aureus
c-ANCA, 135
CBCs. *See* complete blood counts
CCI. *See* corrected count increment
Centers for Disease Control and Prevention (CDC), 198
cerebrospinal fluid (CSF), 198
   gram stain of, 211
cervical lymphadenopathy, 192
chemical hazards, 182–183
children
   coagulation factors in, 87
   protein C, protein S, and antithrombin in, 97
   von Willebrand factor antigen in, 105
Chlamydia, 200
chromoblastomycosis, 205
chronic anemia, rapid transfusion in, 13
chronic myelogenous leukemia (CML), 126
CLIA. *See* Clinical Laboratory Improvement Amendments
clindamycin, 213
clinical chemistry, 143–190
   core chemistry, 146–152
   endocrine testing, 171–175
   laboratory information systems, 175–180
   laboratory safety, 180–185

outreach testing, 185–189
point-of-care testing, 159–171
specimen receiving and processing, 143–146
therapeutic drug monitoring/ toxicology, 152–159
Clinical Laboratory Improvement Amendments (CLIA), 157, 162, 164, 259, 260
   of 1988 law, 161
Clinical Laboratory Standards Institute (CLSI), 221
clinical microbiology
   analytic errors in, 210
   postanalytic errors in, 223–224
   preanalytic errors in, 191
   results, 224–227
clot-based activated protein C resistance assay, 94
CLSI. *See* Clinical Laboratory Standards Institute
CML. *See* chronic myelogenous leukemia
coagulation disorders, 59
coagulation factors
   in children, 87
   deficiencies assessment of, 83–84
coagulation screening test, 2
cold agglutinin disease (CAD), of low antibody titers, 13–14
color-coded tubes, 145
communication breakdowns, 186
Community-associated methicillin-resistant staphylococcus Aureus (CA-MRSA), 203
compensation issues, 272
competitive performance, outreach market, 278–280
competitive products, evaluation of, 282–283
competitive salary, 272

complement testing
   errors in interpretation of, 136
   immunology, 131
complete blood counts
      (CBCs), 121
   measurements, 122
   results, 126
   testing, 122
confirmatory test, 157
   antiphospholipid
         antibodies, 101
congenital hypercoagulable
      state, evaluation for, 93–94
Coombs' test, 29
corrected count increment
      (CCI), 39
Coxiella, 200
CPT code. *See* Current
      Procedural
      Terminology code
critical values, 151, 159
crossmatching blood, 8
cryoglobulins, 139
   errors in analysis of, 139–140
cryoprecipitate, 2
   inappropriate use of, 6–7
crypt antigen activation, 28
cryptococcal antigen test, 211
Cryptococcal meningitis, 201, 210
Cryptococcus, 215
Cryptococcus neoformans, 201
CSF. *See* cerebrospinal fluid
Cumitech series, 210
Current Procedural Terminology
      (CPT) code, 269
CYP2C19, pharmacogenomic
      testing for, 116

DAT. *See* direct antiglobulin test
data analysis, to support
      patient outcomes, 266–267
data collection, to support
      patient outcomes,
      266–267
data entry errors, with patient
      identification, 166

data management systems,
      165, 166
D-dimer tests, 89, 92
delayed hemolytic transfusion
      reactions (DHTRs), 10, 19
delta checks, 121
Department of Transportation
      (DOT) regulations, 183,
      184, 275
DHTRs. *See* delayed hemolytic
      transfusion reactions
diabetes mellitus, 173
diagnostic laboratory
      industry, 282
DIC. *See* disseminated
      intravascular coagulation
DIHA. *See* drug-induced
      hemolytic anemia
diphenhydramine, 37, 38
direct antiglobulin test (DAT), 11
   misinterpretation of, 29–30
direct thrombin inhibitor,
      coagulation factor
      assays, 85
disseminated intravascular
      coagulation (DIC)
   diagnosis of, 90, 91
   evaluation for, 89–90
Donath–Landsteiner test, 24
donor blood, 10
dosing of low molecular weight
      heparin, 72
DOT. *See* Department of
      Transportation
drug-induced hemolytic anemia
      (DIHA), 44–45
drug-induced thrombocytopenia
      assays, 110
drug test, 152
   panels of, 153
dysplasia, 128

ECP. *See* extracorporeal
      photopheresis
ED. *See* emergency department
EDTA, platelet clumping, 111

efficient workflow process, defining, 276
Ehrlichia species, 196
ehrlichiosis, 194
EIA platform. *See* enzyme immunoassay platform
electronic interfaces, 154
electronic medical records (EMRs), 154
ELISA. *See* enzyme-linked immunosorbent assay
emergency department (ED), 152, 154
emergency management, 155
empiric antiviral treatment, 201
employment testing, positive results for, 155
EMRs. *See* electronic medical records
ENAs. *See* extractable nuclear antigens
endocrine testing, 171–175
enzyme immunoassay (EIA) platform, 132
enzyme-linked immunoassays, 79
enzyme-linked immunosorbent assay (ELISA), 198
eosinophilia, 126
eosinophilic leukemia, 126
ethylenediaminetetraacetic acid (EDTA), 122
extracorporeal photopheresis (ECP), 17
extractable nuclear antigens (ENAs), 132, 133

factor VIII inhibitor, 102
  evaluation for, 107–108
FDA. *See* Food and Drug Administration
FDP. *See* fibrinogen degradation products
febrile nonhemolytic transfusion reactions (FNHTRs), 37

ferritin, 124
fetal transfusion, 20
fetomaternal hemorrhage (FMH), 4
fibrinogen, 6, 7
fibrinogen degradation products (FDP), 90
fibronectin, 6
financial management, 268–271
financial reporting tools, 269
FISH. *See* fluorescence in situ hybridization
flow cytometry, 127
fluorescence in situ hybridization (FISH), 126
FMH. *See* fetomaternal hemorrhage
FNHTRs. *See* febrile nonhemolytic transfusion reactions
fondaparinux, anticoagulant therapy monitoring in patients, 72–73
Food and Drug Administration (FDA), 212
food, risks of, 181–182
forensic testing, 152
free light chains, errors in analysis of, 138–139
fresh frozen plasma (FFP), 1–2
  coagulation factor deficiencies with, 86
  to prothrombin time, 1–2
  transfusion of, 1
  for volume expansion, 2–3
  warfarin use of, 30
fuchsin, 213
fungal infections, 193

Gen-Probe Amplified *Mycobacterium tuberculosis* Direct (MTD), 218
Gomori methenamine silver (GMS), 214

gram stain, 213
    misreading or
        misinterpretation of,
        210–216
granulocytic leukocytosis, errors
    in evaluation of, 125–126

half-life for fondaparinux, 74
HDFN. *See* hemolytic
    disease of the fetus and
    newborn
Health Insurance Portability
    and Accountability Act
    (HIPAA) of 1996, 178
hematology
    platelets, 129–131
    preanalytical errors, 121–122
    red blood cells, 122–125
    standards of care, 121–122
    white blood cells, 125–129
hemolysis, 14
    laboratory tests for, 10–11
    platelet transfusion, 15–16
hemolytic anemia, diagnosis
    of, 41
hemolytic complement
    activity, 136
hemolytic disease of the fetus
    and newborn (HDFN),
    3, 19
    diagnosis of, 33–34
hemolytic transfusion reaction,
    10, 26, 43–44
    occult anemia, 18–19
heparin-flushed lines, 17–18
heparin-induced
    thrombocytopenia (HIT),
    17, 64
    argatroban, 77
    evaluation for, 78–80
    fondaparinux, 75
    low molecular weight
        heparin, 69
heparin–platelet factor 4
    complex, 79, 80
    test for antibodies, 81
high risk tests, 266

high volume tests, 266
HIPAA of 1996. *See* Health
    Insurance Portability and
    Accountability Act of 1996
HIT. *See* heparin-induced
    thrombocytopenia
HIT-associated thromboses, 79
HIV infection, 45–46
hyperbilirubinemia, 205
hypercoagulation test, 94
hyperkalemia, RBC transfusion,
    46–47
hypocalcemic toxicity
    symptoms of, 14
    of TPM, 14–15
    treatments of, 15
hypotension, cause of, 35–37
hypotensive transfusion
    reaction, 36

IATA. *See* International Air
    Transport Association
IFA. *See* indirect fluorescence
    assay
IgA deficiency,
    misinterpretations
    and assumptions, 34–35
IgG antibodies.
    See immunoglobulin G
    antibodies
IgM autoantibodies, 13
immature platelet fraction
    (IPF), 130
immune-mediated
    hemolysis in pediatric
    patient, 23–24
immune thrombocytopenia
    (ITP), 130
immunofixation
    electrophoresis, 138
immunoglobulin G (IgG)
    antibodies, 79
immunoglobulins
    cryoglobulins, errors in
        analysis of, 139–140
    free light chains, errors in
        analysis of, 138–139

protein electrophoresis,
        errors in evaluation of,
        137–138
immunology
    autoimmune and
        complement testing, 131
    immunoglobulins, 137–140
indirect fluorescence assay
        (IFA), 132
indwelling catheters,
        collecting samples
        through, 164
infections, 191–194
Infectious Diseases Society of
        America Clinical Practice
        Guidelines, 201
infrastructure requirements,
        279–280
INR value. *See* international
        normalized ratio value
Institute of Medicine report, 261
instrument selection, 282–283
instrument technology,
        acquisition of, 282
International Air Transport
        Association (IATA), 183, 184
international normalized ratio
        (INR) value, 59, 62
    argatroban, 76
international sensitivity index
        (ISI), 61
IPF. *See* immature platelet
        fraction
iron deficiency anemia, 123
ISI. *See* international sensitivity
        index
ITP. *See* immune
        thrombocytopenia

Kleihauer–Betke test, 4, 5

labeling errors, 143–144
laboratory information
        system (LIS), 153, 175–180
    compatability with software
        applications, 285

selection and utilization,
        283–286
staff support for, 284–285
support for, 285
laboratory leadership
    communication, 280
    external resources,
        engaging, 277
    leakage of tests,
        monitoring, 281
    LIS installation,
        managing, 284
    outreach service
        requirements, 279
    performance standards,
        recognizing, 278
    reference laboratories,
        selection of, 280
    responsibility, 263, 266, 268,
        271, 274
    safety standards, 273
    vendors, selection of, 280
laboratory safety, 180–185,
        273–274
laboratory test result report,
        260, 261
Legionella, 201
Legionella bozemanii, 202
Legionella infection, 201
Legionella longbeachae, 202
Legionella micdadei, 202
Legionella pneumophila, 202
length of stay (LOS), 268
Leptospira, 199, 200
leptospirosis, 199
leukoerythroblastic
        reaction, 126
liberal versus restrictive
        transfusion strategies,
        20–21
LIS. *See* laboratory information
        system
liver disease
    confusing DIC with, 90
    PT and PTT in patient
        with, 87
LOS. *See* length of stay

low molecular weight heparin
anticoagulant therapy
monitoring in patients
with, 67–68
platelet count monitoring, 82
lumbar puncture (LP), 21
lung infections, 193
lupus anticoagulant test, 100
clot-based activated protein C
resistance assay, 94
factor VIII inhibitor, 109
screening tests for, 101
systemic lupus
erythematosus, 101
lyme disease, 197, 224
lymphatic tissue, 192
lymph node biopsy, 192
lymphocyte morphology, 127
lymphocytic leukocytosis, errors
in evaluation of, 127

macrothrombocytopenia,
patients with, 130
MAHA. *See* microangiopathic
hemolytic anemia
malaria evaluation, 204
MCV. *See* mean cell volume
MDS. *See* myelodysplastic
syndrome
mean cell volume (MCV), 123
mean platelet volume
(MPV), 130
medical director, 187
medical record, 149
Mentzer index (mCV/RBC), 124
metabolic alkalosis, 47–48
methylene tetrahydrofolate
reductase (MTHFR), 96
MG. *See* myasthenia gravis
microangiopathic hemolytic
anemia (MAHA), 41
microbiology specimen, 203–207
microbiology tests, sensitivity/
specificity, 200–203
microcytic anemia, 123
diagnosis of, 124

microorganism,
misidentification of,
216–221
mild allergic reactions, 38
mistakes, POCT
implementation of, 161–162
ordering, 175–176
quality control, 164–165
sample application, 168–169
test ordering, 162–164
molecular testing, 206
monitor compliance,
273–274
monoclonal
immunoglobulins, 137
mononucleosis-like
syndrome, 226
morphologic dysplasia, 128
MPV. *See* mean platelet
volume
M spike, 137
MTHFR. *See* methylene
tetrahydrofolate reductase
multiple transfusions, 20
myasthenia gravis (MG), 16
Mycobacterium abscessus, 218
Mycoplasma, 200
mycotic infections, 205
myelodysplasia, errors in
diagnosis of, 128
myelodysplastic syndrome
(MDS), 128, 129
myeloma, screening for, 138

nasopharyngeal swabs, 201
National Blood Service
Transfusion
Medicine Clinical Policies
Group, 16
National Committee for Clinical
Laboratory Standards
(NCCLS), 221
neurosyphilis, 225
New Technology
Committee, 188
Nocardia infection, 203

occult anemia, hemolytic
    transfusion reaction, 18–19
Occupational Safety and
    Health Administration
    (OSHA), 180, 273
operating budget reports, 270
operating cost, financial
    impact of, 268
operating expenses, 268
operational processes, 270
opportunity cost, 268
oral contraceptives, 98
oral iron therapy, 124
OSHA, See Occupational Safety
    and Health Administration
osteomyelitis, 205
outreach business model, 185
outreach market
    competitive performance
        in, 278–280
    laboratory services for, 279
    manage staff performance to
        support, 279
outreach testing, 185–189

p-ANCA, 135
panel reactive antibody
    (PRA), 42
partial thromboplastin time
    (PTT), 9
    argatroban, 76
    factor VIII inhibitor, 108
    low molecular weight
        heparin, 68
    prolongations, evaluation
        of, 83–84
    unfractionated heparin,
        63, 65
PAS. See periodic acid-Schiff
passive identification, 262,
    263, 265
patient
    care needs, 282
    failure to identify, 207–210
    identification of, 263–265
    safety, 261–265

PCCs. See prothrombin complex
    concentrates
PCR. See polymerase chain
    reaction
PDGFRA, 126
PDGFRB, 126
Pelger–Huet cells, 128
performance benchmarks, 266
performance improvement,
    265–268
performance standards,
    266–268, 272
performance threshold, 266, 267
periodic acid-Schiff (PAS), 214
peripheral blood smear, 11,
    121–123, 126, 130
pharmacogenomic testing, for
    warfarin sensitivity, 62
Phialophora richardsiae, 205
phlebotomy technique, 149, 151
phosphatidylserine, 100
phospholipid-dependent
    test, 101
photopheresis, 17
plasma, 2
    infusion of, 15
    products, use of, 2, 3
plasmapheresis, 16
platelet clumping, 111, 112
platelet dysfunction, evaluation
    for, 114
platelet-rich plasma, 116
platelets
    counts, 17
    hematology, 129–131
    of cold exposure, 7–8
    refractoriness, evaluation of,
        39–40
    transfusion, 15–16,
        24–25, 49–50
POCT. See point-of-care testing
poikilocytosis, 123
point-of-care testing (POCT),
    159–171, 162
    from central laboratory tests,
        162–163, 169

point-of-care testing (POCT)
(*cont.*)
differences and
limitations, 161
identification numbers,
sharing of, 165
infrequent operators, 169
mistakes. *See* mistakes, POCT
overutilization of, 163–164
reassessing need for, 170
to solve overly complex
system problems, 161
use of, 164
polymerase chain reaction
(PCR), 195, 225
positive ANAs, 132
positive ANCA test, 135
positive DAT, 29, 30
positive patient identification
(PPID), 262, 263, 265
positive RF tests, 134
postanalytical errors
in clinical microbiology,
223–224
core chemistry, 151
endocrine testing, 174
laboratory information
systems, 177–179
outreach testing, 187–188
point-of-care testing,
169–170
therapeutic drug monitoring/
toxicology, 156–158
posttransfusion purpura
(PTP), 25–26
PPID. *See* positive patient
identification
PRA. *See* panel reactive antibody
preanalytical errors
in clinical microbiology, 191
core chemistry, 148–149
endocrine testing, 172–173
hematology, 121–122
laboratory information
systems, 175–176
laboratory safety, 181–184
outreach testing, 186–187

point-of-care testing, 164–166
specimen receiving and
processing, 143–146
pregnancy
alloantibodies in, 19–20
RhIG in, 3–4
premedication for transfusion,
37–39
prenatal care plans, 154
primigravida, alloimmune
thrombocytopenia in,
48–49
procedural shortcuts, 168
product inventory, 270
program opportunities,
assessing, 270–271
prophylactic platelet
transfusion, 49
nonevidence-based practices
in, 21–22
protamine sulfate, 73
protein C
in active clotting, 97
antigenic tests for, 95
in children, 97
deficiency of, 96
patients treated with
warfarin, 94
protein electrophoresis,
errors in evaluation
of, 137–138
protein S
in active clotting, 97
adequacy of, 95
antigenic tests for, 95
in children, 97
deficiency of, 96
low value for, 97
patients treated with
warfarin, 94
prothrombin complex
concentrates (PCCs), 31
prothrombin time (PT)
evaluation of prolongations,
83–84
replacement value for, 62
values, 61

prothrombin time/international normalized ratio (PT/INR), 1
Pseudomonas aeruginosa, 206
pseudo-thrombocytopenia, 111
PT. *See* prothrombin time
PT/INR. *See* prothrombin time/international normalized ratio
PTP. *See* posttransfusion purpura
PTT. *See* partial thromboplastin time
PTT-related coagulation factor assays, 102
pulmonary biopsy specimens, 202

QM program. *See* quality management program
quality control mistakes, 164–165
quality management (QM) program, 265–268

RBC morphology, errors in evaluation of, 122–123
RBCs. *See* red blood cells
reactive lymphocytosis, 127
reagent storage errors, 167–168
recombinant factor VIIa (rFVIIa), 31
red blood cells (RBCs), 4
hematology, 122–125
hyperkalemia, risk of, 46–47
issue of, 8
transfusion, 20
red cell morphologies, 123
red-topped tubes, 148
reference laboratories
monitoring utilization, 280–281
selection and management, 280–282

refractory thrombocytopenia, 39
regulations
DOT, 183, 184, 275
laboratory management, 259–261
state, requirements of, 260
regulatory compliance, 259–261
replacement value for PT, 62
RetHe. *See* reticulocyte hemoglobin
reticulocyte count, errors in interpretation of, 125
reticulocyte hemoglobin (RetHe), 124
revenue management, 269
rFVIIa. *See* recombinant factor VIIa
RhD blood group antigen, alloimmunization to, 4
RhD protein and RhIG, molecular differences in, 22–23
rheumatoid factor test, errors in interpretation of, 134
Rh immune globulin (RhIG)
inadequate dosing, 4–6
in pregnancy, 3–4
Rh-positive RBCs, 4
Rickettsia rickettsii, 196
rickettsiosis, 196
ristocetin cofactor, 105
threshold for, 106
RMSF. *See* Rocky Mountain spotted fever
Roche COBAS AMPLICOR system, 219
Rocky Mountain spotted fever (RMSF), 195
rosette test, 4, 5

safety
laboratory, 273–274
patient, 261–265
safranin, 213
SCD. *See* sickle cell disease

screening tests, 156
  antiphospholipid
    antibodies, 101
  for lupus anticoagulant, 101
sensitivity of microbiology tests,
    200–203
seroconversion of RMSF
    infection, 195
serology tests, 134, 194, 195
  timing for, 198–200
serum free light chains, 139
service requirements, 278, 279
sickle cell disease (SCD),
    alloimmunization in, 26–27
specificity of microbiology tests,
    200–203
specimen
  collection errors, 148–149,
    155–156, 263
  collection tubes, 145
  failure to identify, 207–210
  label, 144
  labeling errors, 144, 149
  logistics, 274–276
  processing errors, 145
  receiving and processing, 143
  storage, 183–184
  transportation, 145, 263,
    275, 276
spirochetes, 199
staffing levels, assessing,
    272, 273
staff management, 271–273
staff performance,
    managing, 279
Staphylococcus lugdunensis, 226
state regulations, requirements
    of, 260
strengths, weaknesses,
    opportunities, and
    threats (SWOT)
    analysis, 278
Streptococcus milleri, 217
Streptococcus pneumoniae, 28, 212
summer flu, 194
supply expenses,
    monitoring, 269

susceptibility testing error,
    221–223
systemic lupus
    erythematosus, 101

TACO. *See* transfusion-
    associated circulatory
    overload
T activation, 28
TAT. *See* turn-around time
temperature monitoring,
    167–168
testing process, adequate
    performance of, 167
test names, 175, 176
test order, failure to identify,
    207–210
test ordering errors, 153–155,
    162–164
test utilization, 276–278
therapeutic drug monitoring,
    152–159
therapeutic plasma exchange
    (TPE), 16–17, 41, 48
  hypocalcemic toxicity, 14–15
Thomsen–Hubener–Friedenrich
    phenomenon, 28
thrombocytopenia, 21, 25, 39,
    41, 205
  errors in evaluation of,
    110, 129
thrombocytosis, errors in
    evaluation of, 130
thrombotic thrombocytopenic
    purpura (TTP), 16, 47, 110
  diagnosis of, 40–42
thyroid-stimulating hormone
    (TSH), 171
tickborne infections, 197
T lymphocytes, blastoid
    transformation of, 197
toxicology testing, 152–159
TRALI. *See* transfusion-related
    acute lung injury
transfusion-associated
    circulatory overload
    (TACO), 13

transfusion medicine
  clinical scenarios errors, 18
  errors in procedures, 8
  product-related errors, 1
transfusion-related acute lung
    injury (TRALI)
  diagnosis of, 42–44
Treponema, 200
TTP. *See* thrombotic
    thrombocytopenic purpura
tuberculosis, 193
tubes, 121
tumor lysis, 131
tumor markers, 171–175
turn-around time (TAT), 266, 267
type I cryoglobulins, 139
type II cryoglobulins, 139
type III cryoglobulins, 140

unfractionated heparin
  anticoagulant therapy
      monitoring in patients
      with, 63–64
  antithrombin assay for
      patient with, 95
  platelet count, 80

vancomycin, 157, 213
vasculitides, 134
VDRL. *See* Venereal Disease
    Research Laboratory
vendors' performance,
    evaluation of, 281

Venereal Disease Research
    Laboratory (VDRL), 225
verbal communication, patient
    identity, 264–265
vital value, 223
vitamin K, 30, 32, 60, 61
volume overload, transfusion
    of chronic anemia
    in, 13
von Willebrand disease,
    evaluation for, 104–106

warfarin, 77
  anticoagulant therapy
      monitoring in patients
      with, 59
  coagulation factor assays, 85
  protein C and protein S
      levels, 94
  reversal of, 30–33
Whipple's disease, diagnosis
    of, 225
white blood cells, hematology
  granulocytic leukocytosis,
      errors in evaluation of,
      125–126
  lymphocytic leukocytosis,
      errors in evaluation
      of, 127
  myelodysplasia, errors in
      diagnosis of, 128
workflow process, defining, 276
workload, assessing, 272, 273

Printed in the United States
By Bookmasters